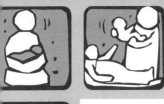

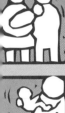
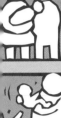

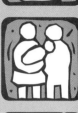

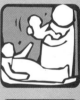

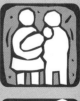

Congratulations on Your Pregnancy

The Department of Defense is proud to welcome you to our Obstetrical Services and will do everything possible to help ensure that you receive the very best prenatal care for both you and your baby. That's why we have implemented Goal-Oriented Prenatal Care.

With goal-oriented care, we design each visit to cover precise goals that are most appropriate to that specific time in your pregnancy. So no matter where you are located in the military system, you will receive all critical aspects of prenatal care at the appropriate time. We have eliminated practices that don't have sound scientific backing (such as taking urine at each visit and early pregnancy cervical checks) and added practices that have been shown to help ensure a healthy pregnancy (such as 20 week ultrasound and fetal movement counts). With this new approach, you will know what to expect and when to expect it.

This book will guide you each step of the way through your pregnancy. We have divided the contents by visits with additional material in alphabetical order in the resource section. Each visit section will include what to expect at your upcoming visit, any additional procedures and labs, signs to report, your weight, blood pressure, uterine growth, baby's heart rate, information on week-related pregnancy concerns, breast-feeding, exercise and diet. We encourage you to read carefully each visit section and related information prior to each appointment. There is space in each visit section to write down questions, record information and take notes as needed. Please ask your health care provider if you have any questions or concerns. In this way, you will be well prepared for each step in this very special journey!

Again, thank you for allowing us to take this journey with you!

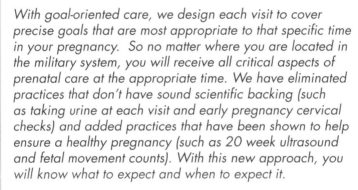

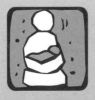
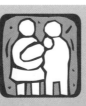
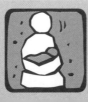

Appointment List				
Date	Time	Provider	Appointment Type	Location
			Initial Labs	Laboratory
			6–8 week visit	
			10–12 week visit	
			Genetic counseling (if indicated)	
			Cystic Fibrosis Carrier Test (if not done prior & desired)	Laboratory
			16–20 week visit	
			Ultrasound (wear loose fitting clothes)	Radiology
			Maternal Serum Analyte Screen (if desired)	
			24 week visit	
			Class sign-up	
			28 week visit	
			Class sign-up	
			28 week labs	
			32 week visit	
			Class sign-up	
			36 week visit	
			Labor & Delivery tour	
			Admission papers to admission office	
			38 week visit	
			39 week visit	
			40 week visit	
			41 week visit	
		Post date testing	NST (twice-weekly)	
			Amniotic fluid check	
			42 week induction	Labor & Delivery

For your Consideration

Goal-oriented visits:

6–8 Week Visit Goal: Exchange information and identify existing risk factors that may impact your pregnancy.

To Do:

1. Read the next visit information and any additional related topics prior to your visit and write down any questions you may have.

2. Ask your family about any medical problems that exist in your family such as diabetes, cancer, hypertension, and genetic problems.

3. Fill out self-administered questionnaire in preparation for this visit.

4. Suggested reading: the Cystic Fibrosis Carrier Test and HIV consent forms and think about whether you wish to have these blood tests performed.

10–12 Week Visit Goal: Determine current health status and work towards a healthy pregnancy.

To Do:

1. Read the visit information and any additional related topics prior to your visit and write down any questions you may have.

2. Wear easy to change out of clothing for physical exam.

3. Suggested reading: "Common Discomforts and Annoyances of Pregnancy" and Maternal Serum Analyte Screen consent form both found in the Resource Section of this booklet for next visit (16-20 week) and think about whether you wish to have this blood test performed.

16–20 Week Visit Goal: Work towards a more comfortable & safer pregnancy.

To Do:

1. Read the visit information and any additional related topics prior to your visit and write down any questions you may have.

2. Allow time for Ultrasound if scheduled with this appointment.

24-Week Visit Goal: Prevent Pre-term Labor for a safe and healthy baby.

To Do:

1. Read the visit information and any additional related information prior to your visit and write down any questions and concerns you may have.

2. Suggested reading: "Pre-Term Labor" found in the 24-Week Visit Chapter of this booklet and local listing of classes found in the Clinic and Hospital Section of this booklet.

28-Week Visit Goal: Monitor your baby and your progress and learn to count fetal movements.

To Do:

1. Read the visit information and any additional related topics prior to your visit and write down any questions and concerns you may have.

2. Follow instructions given to you for your 1-hour glucola test.

3. Suggested reading: "Fetal Movement Counts" under "Testing and Monitoring" found in the Resource Section of this booklet.

32-Week Visit Goal: Prepare for your baby's arrival.

To Do:

1. Read the visit information and any additional related topics prior to your visit and write down any questions or concerns you may have.

2. Fill out Fetal Movement Chart and bring with you to visit.

3. Suggested reading: "Labor and Delivery" found in the Resource Section of this booklet.

36-Week Visit Goal: Begin preparations for your hospital experience.

To Do:

1. Read the visit information and any additional related topics prior to your visit and write down any questions and concerns you may have.

2. Fill out Fetal Movement Chart and bring with you to visit.

3. Suggested reading: "Labor and Delivery" found in the Resource Section of this booklet.

38–41 Week Visit Goal: Preparing for the delivery and baby's arrival at home.

To Do:

1. Read the visit information and any additional related topics prior to your visit and write down any questions or concerns you may have.

2. Fill out Fetal Movement Chart and bring with you to visit.

3. Suggested reading: "Postdate Pregnancy Plan" found in the 38–41-Week Visit Chapter and "Baby Equipment for the First Week" found in the Resource Section of this booklet.

Resource Section:

- **Consent Forms**
    - Cystic Fibrosis Carrier Screen
    - Human Immunodeficiency Virus (HIV)
    - Maternal Serum Analyte Screen

- **Pregnancy Information**
    - Active Duty Information
    - Anatomy (front & side views)
    - Common Discomforts and Annoyances of Pregnancy
    - Fetal Movement Count Charts (5 total)
    - Immunizations
    - Nutrition in Pregnancy
        Food Guide Pyramid
        BMI Chart
        Weight Gain Chart
    - Sexually Transmitted Diseases, Infections, & Pregnancy
    - Testing and Monitoring During Pregnancy
    - True versus False Labor

- **Labor & Delivery**
    - Labor & Delivery Basics
    - Birth Plan

- **After The Delivery**
    - Baby Equipment
    - Birth Control
    - Breast-Feeding
    - Bottle Feeding
    - Safety Tips for Baby

- **Common Terms**

- **Types of Providers**

Suggested Additional Readings (available in your clinic):

- Birth defects (ACOG Pamphlet 146)
- Cystic Fibrosis Carrier Testing: The Decision is Yours
- Cystic Fibrosis Testing: What Happens if Both My Partner and I are Carriers?
- Group B Streptococcus and Pregnancy (ACOG Pamphlet 105)
- Having Twins (ACOG Pamphlet 092)
- High Blood Pressure During Pregnancy (ACOG Pamphlet 034)
- HIV Testing and Pregnancy (ACOG Pamphlet 113)
- Illegal Drugs & Pregnancy (ACOG Pamphlet 104)
- Maternal Serum Screening for Birth Defects (ACOG Pamphlet 089)
- Prenatal Fitness and Exercise
- Pre-Term Labor (ACOG Pamphlet 087)
- Sterilization for Women and Men (ACOG Pamphlet 011)
- The Rh Factor: How it can Affect Your Pregnancy (ACOG Pamphlet 027)
- What to Expect After Your Due Date (ACOG Pamphlet 069)

Web sites:

http://www.nlm.nih.gov/medlineplus/ (general pregnancy and health)
http://www.healthfinder.gov (general pregnancy and health)
http://www.modimes.org/ (general pregnancy, baby and health)
http://familydoctor.org/ (general pregnancy, baby and health)
http://mama.modimes.org/ (general pregnancy,baby and health)
http://www.childbirth.org/ (childbirth)
http://www.4women.org/ (women's health,nutrition and birth control)
http://www.lalecheleague.org/ (breast-feeding)
http://www..plannedparenthood.org (birth control)
http://www.gotmom.org (breast-feeding)
http://healtheforces.org (military and health care)
http://www.asahq.org/patientEducation/childbirth.pdf (options for pain relief during labor)

6–8 Weeks Visit Prenatal Information Sheet

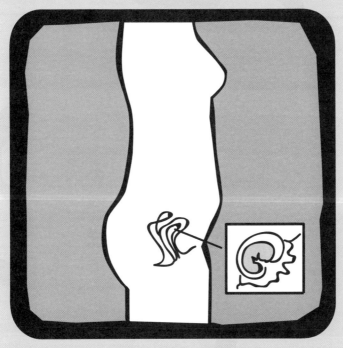

Goal: Exchange information and identify existing risk factors that may impact the pregnancy.

Prenatal Information Sheet: *6–8 Weeks Visit*

Goal: Exchange information and identify existing risk factors that may impact the pregnancy.

Today's visit

- If possible, prior to this visit, fill out self-administered questionnaire about your history that is relevant to this pregnancy.
- Screen for your potential risk factors such as:
  - **Social risks:** alcohol/drug/tobacco/domestic abuse
  - **Medical risks:** immunization status, exposure to sexually transmitted diseases, current health status, and family history of specific diseases
  - **Nutritional risks:** weight and dietary intake
  - **Obstetrical risks:** problems in previous pregnancies and risks for pre-term labor
- If you are struggling with nausea and vomiting, refer to the table, "Common Discomforts & Annoyances of Pregnancy" in the Resource Section for things you can do. Now is the time to also think about avoiding too much weight gain. Refer to the "Nutrition in Pregnancy" section in the Resource Section for tips to avoid too much weight gain.
- Receive and discuss information on exercise, benefits of breast-feeding, and other health related behaviors.
- Receive education and counseling on pregnancy laboratory tests to include Cystic Fibrosis Carrier and Rh factor screening, anemia, and others.
- Receive needed immunizations and information on ways to decrease chance of getting various diseases.
- Have recommended blood work and urine screen completed.
- Discuss your anticipated due date which may change when more information is known and further testing is done.

Today's visit

Your baby's growth

- Your baby (embryo) is an inch long and weighs 1/30 of an ounce.
- Your baby's face and body are fairly well formed.
- Your baby's bones have appeared, internal organs are beginning to work, and the baby's heart has been beating since the third week.

Your baby's growth

continued next page

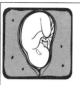

Your baby's growth

Your baby's growth (cont.)

- The placenta is attached to the uterine (womb) wall on the mother's side and the umbilical cord going to the baby on the other. The placenta acts as an "almost" perfect filtering system between mother's blood and baby's blood. The placenta has a fetal (baby) circulation side and the maternal circulation side. A membrane barrier separates these sides. It is the placenta and umbilical cord that provides a way for the nutrients (food and oxygen) to get to your baby and for waste products to be removed. Unfortunately, it also allows some harmful substances, such as alcohol, if in the mother's blood, to get to the baby as well.

Your body's changes

Your body's changes

- Your uterus has grown from the size of a pear to the size of a large orange.
- You are probably beginning to notice changes in your body as a result of your pregnancy.
- Your breasts may become larger and tender.
- The area around your nipples may darken.
- You may have to go to the bathroom more frequently to urinate.
- You may have morning sickness that lasts beyond morning.
- Your bowel habits may change with increased constipation.

Your family's changes

Your family's changes

- The hormone changes that affect your body may also effect your emotions, causing mood swings.
- Your partner may have concerns about your health, the baby, and your financial state.
- Coping with the discomforts of pregnancy may change household and work routines.
- You both need time to adjust and accept your upcoming role as new or repeat parents.
- It is important to share these feelings with someone you trust.

Signs to report immediately

Signs to report immediately

- Bright red vaginal bleeding, gush of fluid from the vagina and/or four or more painful cramping contractions within an hour (after resting and emptying bladder).
- Persistent severe headaches, severe nausea, and vomiting.
- Fever over 100.5° F or 38° C.
- Inability to keep liquids down resulting in a reduced amount of urine.
- When in doubt, call the clinic or your healthcare provider!

Notes:	Discussion:	Key points:

Normal is same as pre-pregnant BP or slightly less than pre-pregnant BP.

My BP:

_____

Your blood pressure

- We will measure blood pressure (BP) at every prenatal visit. Rapidly increasing or abnormally high blood pressure can be a sign of Pregnancy Induced Hypertension (PIH).
- High blood pressure can cause serious complications such as a decrease in the blood and oxygen supply to the baby and mother.

Your blood pressure

My weight:

_____

Your weight

- You are likely to gain 2 to 4 pounds in the first three months.
- Total weight gain should be about 25 pounds unless you are over or underweight. Your weight gain is not all fat. It is mostly water in your body and the weight of the growing baby.
- Normal pregnancy weight gain: (If pre-pregnant BMI is normal)

Your weight

breast	1.0 - 1.5 lbs.
blood	3.0 - 4.5 lbs.
extra water	4.0 - 6.0 lbs.
uterus	2.5 - 3.0 lbs.
placenta/amniotic fluid	3.5 lbs.
baby	7.0 - 8.0 lbs.
fat stores	4.0 - 6.5 lbs.
TOTAL	**25 - 35 lbs.**

- Gaining the right amount of weight by eating the right type of food is an extremely important part of a healthy pregnancy.

Reference: Prenatal Fitness and Exercise

Your exercise routine

- Regular exercise helps you to keep fit during your pregnancy and to feel better during a time when your body is changing.
- Before beginning a new type of exercise, check with your health care provider.

Your exercise routine

Consider breast-feeding

- Now is the time to think about how you want to feed your baby.
- The American Academy of Pediatrics, the American College of Nurse-Midwives, the American College of OB/GYN, and the American Dietetic Association all strongly recommend breast-feeding for at least your baby's first 12 months of life.

Consider breast-feeding

Take only medications approved by your health care provider

- Safe over-the-counter drugs for common discomforts (If you are less than 12 weeks, discuss all medication use first with your provider.):
  - Headaches: Tylenol®, Datril®
  - Cold: Tylenol®, Sudafed®, Saline nose spray, Robitussin® (no alcohol)
  - Constipation: Metamucil®, Fiber-All®, Milk of Magnesia®
  - Diarrhea: Kaopectate®
  - Indigestion: Tums®, Rolaids®, Maalox®, Mylanta II® and Riopan®
  - Hemorrhoids: Preparation H®, Anusol®
  - Nausea/Vomiting: Vitamin B6 (up to 75mg day), Emetrol®, Unisom®

Take only medications approved by your provider

Drugs to avoid

- Aspirin®, Motrin®/Ibuprofen, Tetracycline, Accutane®
- Caffeine may cause problems with your pregnancy.
- Alcohol, tobacco, and any illicit drugs are harmful to your baby, avoidance helps decrease risks.
- If you are using any drugs or substances that may be harmful to your baby, ask about strategies to quit and approaches to lifestyle behavior changes.

Drugs to avoid

Resource: Illegal Drugs and Pregnancy (ACOG Pamphlet AP 104)

Notes:	Discussion:	Key points:

Work and household activities

- AVOID:
  - Cat litter
  - X-rays (may be necessary after discussion with your OB health care provider)
  - Use of dry cleaning solutions
  - Acrylic nail manicures
  - Children's sandboxes
  - Working around radiation or radioisotopes
  - Working with lead or mercury
  - Gardening without gloves
- If in doubt about your potential exposures, ask your health care provider.

Work and household activities

Reference:
HIV Testing and Pregnancy (ACOG Pamphlet 113)

Contact with certain diseases

- Sexually Transmitted Diseases (STDs) are viruses, or bacteria, or parasites that pose risks or possible death to your baby. It is important that you be honest with your health care provider. These STDs include:
  - HIV(AIDS)
  - Gonorrhea
  - Syphilis
  - Chlamydia
  - Genital Herpes
  - Genital warts

Contact with certain diseases

Immunization status

- Check immunization history and/or past exposure to include:
  - Varicella (Chicken Pox)
  - Rubella (German Measles)
  - Hepatitis B
  - Tetanus: (Lockjaw)
  - Influenza (Flu) (seasonal-related)
- Receive immunizations as needed.

Immunization status

**Domestic abuse
screen**

Domestic abuse screen

- Please seek help from your health care provider, counselor or close friend if you are experiencing physical, sexual, or emotional abuse.
- Let your health care provider know if:
  - Within the last year, or since you have been pregnant, you have been hit, slapped, kicked, otherwise physically hurt, or forced to have sexual activities.
- National Domestic Abuse Hotline: 1-800-799-7233.

Summary of visit

Summary of visit

Due date: _____

Date of next visit: _____

Date for lab work/other medical tests:

_____

Your next visit

Your next visit

- Bring your outpatient medical record and shot record for your provider to review and complete your medical history.
- Receive complete head-to-toe physical and pelvic exam including a Pap smear and cultures for Gonorrhea and Chlamydia.
- Discuss lab test results from first visit and have additional labs if needed.
- Discuss lifestyle changes if needed.
- Receive further education on Cystic Fibrosis Carrier risk and discuss your options to be screened with a blood test if not done on first visit.
- **Every visit:** We will measure your uterine growth, blood pressure, weight, listen to the fetal heart rate (can't always hear this early in pregnancy), and discuss any concerns/ questions you may have.
- Plan on at least a thirty minute visit with your provider.

Questions for next visit

❏ _____

❏ _____

Questions for next visit

❏ _____

❏ _____

❏ _____

Further information on the topics covered in this visit can be found at the end of the notebook.

Listing of medications/drugs does not represent endorsement by VA/DoD

10–12 Weeks Visit Prenatal Information Sheet

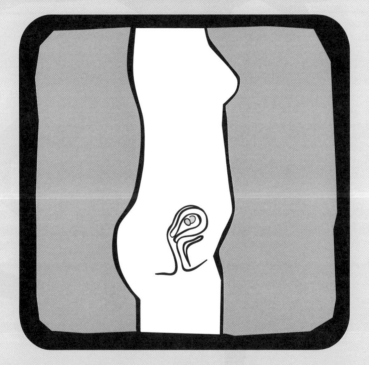

Goal: Determine your current health status and work towards a healthy pregnancy.

Prenatal Information Sheet: 10–12 Weeks Visit

Goal: Determine your current health status and work towards a healthy pregnancy.

Today's visit

- Review medical history.
- Receive complete head-to-toe physical and pelvic exam including a Pap smear and cultures for Gonorrhea and Chlamydia.
- Obtain height and weight to determine amount of fat in your body called the Body Mass Index (BMI).
- Review and discuss initial lab results.
- Receive further testing, counseling, and referral for possible inherited diseases (includes Cystic Fibrosis Carrier screen today, and Maternal Serum Analyte Screen at 15-20 weeks.

Today's visit

Your baby's growth

- Your baby (embryo) is about 2.5 to 3.0 inches long and weighs about 0.5 ounces.
- During this time, your baby's body and organ tissues grow rapidly.
- The head is about twice the size of the body.
- The eyes and ears are moving into normal positions.
- Intestines move from the umbilical cord into the stomach area.
- We may be able to hear your baby's heartbeat with a Doppler.

Your baby's growth

Your body's changes

- Your uterus is now the size of a grapefruit.
- We may be able to feel the upper edge of your uterus (the fundus) a little bit above your pubic bone.
- Wear comfortable clothing that provides room to grow.
- Morning sickness often diminishes by the end of this month (but not always).
- If you haven't already started, slowly add healthier food choices and change unhealthy eating habits to become a positive role model for your baby.

Your body's
changes

Your family's changes

- You may be moody, irritable, tearful, disorganized, have trouble concentrating, or have irrational thoughts. These feelings are normal.
- Unfortunately, this mental "fog" may not lift until after your baby begins sleeping through the night.
- Accept how you're feeling and remember that these feelings will be temporary.
- Your sexual desire may increase or decrease; both are normal.
- Discuss these feelings with others.

Your family's
changes

Signs to report
immediately

Signs to report immediately

- Bright red vaginal bleeding, gush of fluid from the vagina, and/or four or more painful cramping contractions within an hour (after resting and emptying bladder).
- Persistent severe headaches, severe nausea, and vomiting.
- Fever over 100.5° F or 38° C.
- Inability to keep liquids down resulting in a reduced amount of urine.
- When in doubt, call the clinic or your health care provider!

Notes:	Discussion:	Key points:
My BP: _____	**Your blood pressure** • Blood pressure is measured at every prenatal visit because high blood pressure can cause serious complications for baby and mother if left unchecked.	**Your blood pressure**
My weight: _____	**Your weight** • Weight gain by now is usually 2 to 4 pounds. • Your baby is likely to be healthier if you eat nutritious foods. • Try small, frequent meals to provide needed nutrition and to decrease nausea and vomiting. • Choose your calories wisely—make sure each one is good for both the baby and you.	**Your weight** '
Reference: Prenatal Fitness and Exercise	**Your exercise routine** • You may become short of breath even when walking upstairs. Take it slowly. • It is best to never exercise to the point of exhaustion or breathlessness. This is a sign that your body cannot get the oxygen supply it needs, which affects the oxygen supply to the baby as well. • Avoid exercises that involve low oxygen environments, such as scuba diving or mountain climbing.	**Your exercise**
	Consider breast-feeding • Get to know other breast-feeding moms and get involved in community breast-feeding groups, such as La Leche League. • Human breast milk contains over 100 protective ingredients not found in a cow's milk-based formula and breast milk can't be duplicated. • Learn as much about breast-feeding as you can ahead of time.	**Consider breast-feeding**
Fetal heart rate: _____	**Fetal heart rate** • You may be able to hear your baby's heartbeat at this time with a Doppler.	**Fetal heart rate**

Key points:	Discussion:	Notes:
Fundal height	**Fundal height** • Your uterus is measured from your pubic bone to the fundus to check growth of your baby. The height of the uterus in centimeters usually equals the number of weeks pregnant. • At 10-12 weeks your uterus is at the top of your pubic bone.	Fundal height: _____
Initial lab results	**Initial lab results** • If any of your test results are abnormal, your provider will discuss life-style changes, treatments, and possible outcomes.	

Rh (D) Factor screen	**Rh (D) Factor screen**
	 • Rh blood typing and antibody testing will tell if you are Rh (D) negative or positive.
	 • If you are found to be Rh (D) negative:
	   – You will receive a D-immunoglobulin (RhoGAM) shot at 28 weeks to prevent your blood from building up antibodies that can harm your baby.
	   – The D-immunoglobulin (RhoGAM) shot will be given if you have certain procedures, such as aminocentesis, or if you are experiencing vaginal bleeding during the pregnancy.
	   – The D-immunoglobulin (RhoGAM) shot is repeated after delivery if baby's blood is Rh positive.
		Resource: The Rh Factor: How It Can Affect Your Pregnancy (ACOG Pamphlet AP 027)

Rubella and Varicella results	**Rubella and Varicella results** • If screening shows no immunity (tests negative), we will discuss precautions to protect against these infections.	

Asymptomatic Bacteruria screen

- ASB is an increased growth of bacteria in the urine that can only be found through laboratory analysis. There are no symptoms, but ASB can result in a serious kidney infection if left untreated.
- Antibiotic treatment may be prescribed. It is important to take as directed and finish the whole prescription or the bacteria can return.
- To reduce the chance of getting ASB, wear cotton panties and wipe from front to back.

Asymptomatic
Bacteruria (ASB)
screen

Resource:
Cystic Fibrosis
Carrier
Testing: The
Decision Is
Yours and
Cystic Fibrosis
Testing: What
Happens
if Both My
Partner and I
are Carriers
(ACOG
Pamphlets)

Cystic Fibrosis (CF) Carrier Screen

- We offer this test to determine if you are a carrier for CF and your baby's chances of having the disease. If you test positive, then we will want to test the baby's father.
- If you and your partner are carriers, your unborn baby will have a 1 in 4 (25%) chance of having CF.
- You will be given additional information, a CF Carrier Screen consent form and the option for further counseling.
- This information allows couples to decide on their options.
- This test is optional. The chances of having CF vary with ethnic groups.

Cystic Fibrosis
(CF) carrier screen

Your libido

- In early pregnancy, you may find that your desire for sex decreases (especially if you have nausea, vomiting, fatigue, or breast tenderness).
- Since the amniotic sac normally protects and cushions the baby, intercourse normally does not hurt the baby or cause a miscarriage.

Your libido

Your next visit

- **Every visit:** We will measure your uterine growth, blood pressure, weight, listen to your baby's heart rate, and discuss concerns/ questions you may have.
- Schedule Maternal Serum Analyte Screen if desired.

Your next visit

continued next page

Key points:	Discussion:	Notes:

	Your next visit (cont.)	
Your next visit	• Follow-up results of Cystic Fibrosis Carrier Screen if done. • Schedule Ultrasound during the 16–20 week timeframe, so wear clothes that will expose your abdomen easily.	
Questions for next visit	**Questions for next visit** ❑ _____ ❑ _____ ❑ _____ ❑ _____ ❑ _____	

Further information on the topics covered in this visit can be found at the end of the notebook.

Listing of medications/drugs does not represent endorsement by VA/DoD

16–20 Weeks Visit Prenatal Information Sheet

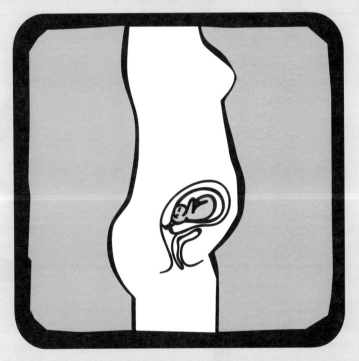

Goal: Work towards a more comfortable and safer pregnancy.

Prenatal Information Sheet: 16–20 Weeks Visit

Goal: Work towards a more comfortable and safer pregnancy.

Today's visit

- **Every visit:** We will measure your uterine growth, blood pressure, weight, listen to baby's heart rate, and discuss any concerns/questions you may have.
- Receive Maternal Serum Analyte Screen, if desired.
- Have an Ultrasound.
- Discuss how to identify differences in pre-term labor versus false labor.

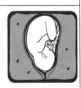

Today's visit

Your baby's growth

- Your baby is now about 4.4 to 5.5 inches long and weighs about 4 ounces.
- Fine hair, called "lanugo," is growing on your baby's head and is starting to cover the body. Fingernails are well-formed.
- The arms and legs are moving and you may start feeling this movement. This movement is called "quickening." You may not feel movement everyday at this point, but the movements will become stronger and more frequent as your pregnancy progresses.

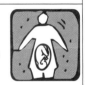

Your baby's growth

Your body's changes

- Your uterus is about the size of a cantaloupe.
- Your center of gravity changes as your uterus grows. This change may affect your balance and your ability to move.
- There is an increase in the mobility of your joints that can affect your posture and cause discomfort in your lower back. As your uterus grows, the round ligaments supporting the uterus can stretch and pull. This ligament pain feels like a sharp pulling sensation on either or both sides of the lower abdomen.
- Some women may have difficulty sleeping.
- Some women complain of head stuffiness or frequent nose bleeds. These symptoms may occur because of changes in your circulatory system due to hormone changes.
- You may notice a whitish, vaginal discharge.
- Constipation may be a problem. Refer to the table, "Common Discomforts & Annoyances of Pregnancy" in the Resource Section for things you can do.

Your body's changes

Your family's changes

- Now is the time to begin discussing birth control with your partner and health care provider. There are many effective options available for you.
- Keep in mind that breast-feeding alone is not a very effective birth control method and that many methods can also be used safely while breast-feeding.

Your family's changes

Signs to report immediately

Signs to report immediately

- Bright red vaginal bleeding, gush of fluid from the vagina and/or four or more painful cramping contractions within an hour (after resting and emptying bladder).
- Persistent severe headaches, severe nausea, and vomiting.
- Fever over 100.5° F or 38° C.
- Inability to keep liquids down resulting in a reduced amount of urine.
- When in doubt, call the clinic or your health care provider!

Notes:	Discussion:	Key points:

My BP:
_____

Your blood pressure

• Report these symptoms: headache, blurred vision, sudden weight gain, swelling of hands and face, and decreased urination.

Your blood pressure

My weight:
_____

Your weight

• The usual weight gain is approximately one pound a week during the rest of the pregnancy.
• Water contributes to 62% of the weight gain, fat 30% and protein 8%.
• Slow and steady weight gain is best.
• Use your chart to monitor your rate of weight gain.
• Severely limit or avoid alcohol completely. No amount of alcohol is safe for your baby.

Your weight

Reference: Prenatal Fitness and Exercise

Your exercise routine

• Stay off your back while exercising from now on.
• Mental, emotional and social benefits of exercise include:
  – Helping to prevent depression
  – Promoting relaxation and restful sleep
  – Encouraging concentration and improving problem solving
  – Helping prepare for childbirth and parenting
  – Helping prevent excess weight gain
  – Improving self-esteem and well being

Your exercise

Consider breast-feeding

• Some advantages to baby include:
  – Easier digestion of breast milk
  – No allergy problems to breast milk
  – Less likely to cause overweight babies
  – Less constipation
  – Easier on baby's kidneys
  – Fewer illnesses in the first year of life
  – Less SIDS (Sudden Infant Death Syndrome)
  – Close contact with mom

Consider breast-feeding

Key points:	Discussion:	Notes:
 **Fetal heart rate**	**Fetal heart rate** • Usually your baby's heartbeat is easier to locate and hear at this time in your pregnancy.	Fetal heart rate: _____
Fundal height	**Fundal height** • At 16 weeks, your uterus is usually midway between the belly button and the pubic bone or 16 cm above the pubic bone. • Beginning at 20 weeks, the fundal height in centimeters will be about equal to the number of weeks you are pregnant.	Fundal height: _____
 **Maternal Serum Analyte Screen**	**Maternal Serum Analyte Screen** • The Maternal Serum Analyte Screen gives you an idea of your risk for having a baby with certain types of genetic defects such as Down's Syndrome or spina bifida (opening around the spine). Most babies (97%) are born without any major defects. • Birth defects may result from viruses, exposure to harmful substances (drugs, chemicals), inherited (genes passed down) from the parents or unknown causes. • If the test results are elevated, it may be due to reasons other than your baby's condition and further testing will be required. • We recommend the decision to undergo this screening but it is optional.	Resource: Maternal Serum Screening for Birth Defects (ACOG Pamphlet AP 089)
"False Labor"	**"False Labor"** • Braxton-Hicks contractions or "False Labor" are usually painless, irregular uterine contractions or tightening of the uterus that begin as early as your sixth week of pregnancy in preparation for labor. • Most women, especially if it's their first pregnancy, will not feel any contractions until after 20 weeks. • Towards the end of pregnancy these contractions increase in frequency, duration, and intensity and are often confused with true labor. • If you are not sure what you are feeling, ask your health care provider.	

Ultrasound

- A painless test in which pictures (called sonograms) of the fetus are made from sound waves. A trained technician will do the ultrasound exams. Wear clothes that allow your abdomen to be exposed easily.

Ultrasound

- An ultrasound provides information about your baby's health and well being inside the womb such as:
  - Age
  - The number of babies
  - Rate of growth
  - Placenta position
  - Baby's heart rate
  - Amount of amniotic fluid
  - Some birth defects
  - Sex
- **Please note:** If you do not wish to know your baby's sex, let the technician know prior to the exam. It may not be possible or 100% accurate to determine the sex by Ultrasound.

Summary of visit

Due date: _____

Blood test results: _____

Date of next visit: _____

Summary of visit

Date for lab work/other medical tests:

_____

Your next visit

- **Every visit:** We will measure your uterine growth, blood pressure, weight, listen to your baby's heart rate, and discuss any concerns/questions you may have.

Your next visit

Questions for next visit

Questions for next visit

❑ _____

❑ _____

❑ _____

❑ _____

❑ _____

Further information on the topics covered in this visit can be found at the end of the notebook.

24 Weeks Visit Prenatal Information Sheet

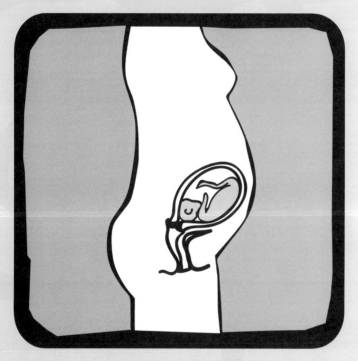

Goal: Prevent pre-term labor for a safe
and healthy baby.

Prenatal Information Sheet: *24 Weeks Visit*

Goal: Prevent pre-term labor for a safe and healthy baby.

Today's visit

Today's visit

- **Every visit:** We will measure your uterine growth, blood pressure, weight, listen to your baby's heart rate, and discuss any concerns/questions you may have.
- Schedule lab tests.
- Sign up for breast-feeding classes and others.
- Check to see if you are having any pre-term labor.
- Learn the signs of pre-term labor and what to do if it occurs.

Your baby's growth

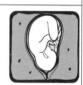

Your baby's growth

- Your baby is now about 8.4 inches long and weighs about 1.2 pounds.
- Your baby is resting and growing inside your uterus, inside of an amniotic sac filled with fluid. This sac provides the perfect environment for your baby. Movement is easy and the sac serves as a cushion for the fetus against injury. The fluid in the sac also regulates the temperature. The fluid level should now begin to increase steadily.

Your body's changes

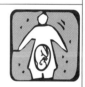

Your body's changes

- Your uterus is now an inch or two above the belly button and is about the size of a small soccer ball.
- You may feel an occasional tightening of your abdomen (Braxton-Hicks), which is normal.
- You may develop varicose veins, increasing heartburn, and skin changes due to the fluctuation in hormones.
- If you have any of the signs of pre-term labor, such as cramping or contractions that do not go away within an hour of rest, call your provider immediately.

Your family's changes

Your family's changes

- Talk to your family about ways to help each other adjust to the many changes you are all facing. Encourage their involvement by inviting them to your clinic visits. Jointly plan for the future and share the many emotions, fears, and joys you are all going through. The more your family is involved now, the easier they will bond with the new baby and participate in his/her care.
- If the father is of the baby is not available, find someone you trust and who is willing to be your support person.

Signs to report
immediately

Signs to report immediately

- Bright red vaginal bleeding, gush of fluid from the vagina, and/ or four or more painful cramping contractions within an hour (after resting and emptying bladder).
- Persistent severe headaches, severe nausea and vomiting.
- Fever over 100.5° F or 38° C.
- Visual changes such as bright white spots or loss of sight.
- Inability to keep liquids down resulting in a reduced amount of urine.
- When in doubt, call the clinic or your health care provider!

Notes	Discussion	Key points
My BP: _____	**Your blood pressure** • Report symptoms such as: headache, blurred vision, sudden weight gain, swelling of hands and face, and decreased urination.	Your blood pressure
My weight: _____	**Your weight** • Your weight gain may be highest during the second trimester averaging closer to 1 ½ pounds gained per week. • Many common discomforts of pregnancy (constipation, nausea, heartburn) can be reduced through a change in diet. • Make sure to get 2 servings of citrus fruits containing Vitamin C each day.	Your weight
Reference: Prenatal Fitness and Exercise	**Your exercise routine** • We recommend that you add 100 to 200 calories to your diet and a full glass of water for every 30 minutes of exercise you do. • The American College of OB/GYN advises women to avoid bouncing, jumping, jarring or high-impact motions. • Always check with your health care provider before beginning a new exercise.	Your exercise

	Consider breast-feeding
	
	• Some advantages of breast-feeding to you include:
	  – Uses 200 to 300 calories each day that allows you to use up some of the extra fat you have stored during your pregnancy.
	  – Helps your uterus get back to its normal size faster.
	  – Saves time, money and extra trips to the store for formula and supplies.
	• There are no special foods you have to eat; however, you should eat a well-balanced diet, and limit alcohol and caffeine.
		Consider breast-feeding

<table>
<tr><td>

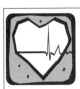

Fetal heart rate

</td><td>

Fetal heart rate

• Baby's heartbeat is getting much easier to hear.

</td><td>

Fetal heart rate:

_____

</td></tr>
<tr><td>

Fundal height

</td><td>

Fundal height

• Fundal height is about 24 cm or 2 inches above the belly button.

</td><td>

Fundal height:

_____

</td></tr>
<tr><td>

Pre-term labor guidelines

</td><td>

Pre-term labor guidelines

• Your baby needs to continue to grow inside you for the full term of your pregnancy. Labor earlier than three weeks before your due date can lead to a premature (preemie) baby with many associated risks.

• **Report to your health care provider any of the following symptoms:**

  – Low, dull backache

  – Four or more uterine contractions per hour. Uterine contractions may be perceived by you as:

    ▪ Menstrual cramps

    ▪ Sensation of the "baby rolling up in a ball"

    ▪ Abdominal cramping (may be associated with diarrhea)

    ▪ Increased uterine activity compared to previous patterns

  – Increased pelvic pressure (may be with thigh cramps)

  – Sensation that "something feels different" (e.g., agitation, flu-like syndrome, and sensation that baby has "dropped").

• **If you experience any of the above symptoms you should:**

  – Stop what you are doing and empty your bladder.

  – Drink 3-4 glasses of water.

</td><td>

Resource: Pre-Term Labor (ACOG Pamphlet AP 087)

</td></tr>
</table>

Notes:	Discussion:	Key points:

Pre-term labor guidelines (cont.)

Pre-term labor guidelines (cont.)

– Lie down on your left side for one hour and place your hands on your abdomen and feel for tightening and hardening of your uterus.

– Count how many contractions you have in an hour.

– If you have more than four contractions in an hour call either the clinic or Labor & Delivery immediately.

• You should report immediately:

– Change in vaginal discharge such as change in color of mucus, leaking of clear fluid, spotting or bleeding, or a vaginal discharge with a fish-like odor immediately after intercourse.

Domestic abuse screen

Domestic abuse screen

• Abuse often begins or increases during pregnancy. The abuse may be physical, sexual or emotional abuse. If the abuse is physical, such as blows to the abdomen, the fetus is at danger for direct injury, miscarriage and/or low birth weight.

• Please seek help from your health care provider, counselor or close friend.

• National Domestic Abuse Hotline: 1-800-799-7233

Key points:	Discussion:	Notes:

Gestational Diabetes (GD) testing

- You will receive a blood test for gestational diabetes. This blood test will tell how your body is responding to your sugar levels.
- Gestational diabetes is abnormal sugar levels in your blood during your pregnancy. It usually goes away after delivery. If your results are high, this does not mean you have diabetes, it just means further testing is needed.
- To prepare for the test at your next visit, eat your usual dinner the night before the test and your normal breakfast the day of the test.
- At the lab, you will be given a glass of glucola to drink which is a very sweet drink that has a specific amount of sugar in it.
- During the hour between drinking the glucola and having your blood drawn, do not eat or drink anything except water, including gum and candy, because they may affect the test results.

Summary of visit

Date of next visit: _____

Date for lab work/other medical tests:

_____

Your next visit

- **Every visit:** We will measure your uterine growth, blood pressure, weight, listen to your baby's heart rate, and discuss any concerns/ questions you may have.
- Receive instructions on counting fetal movement.
- Receive RhoGAM® (D-immunoglobulin) if your blood is Rh negative (D-) and you are not sensitized.
- Have blood work for gestational diabetes and other labs if needed. You will have to wait one hour between drinking the glucola and having your blood drawn.
- Sign up for breast-feeding and other available classes.

Questions for next visit

❏ _____

❏ _____

❏ _____

❏ _____

❏ _____

Questions for next visit

Further information on the topics covered in this visit can be found at the end of the notebook.

Listing of medications/drugs does not represent endorsement by VA/DoD

28 Weeks Visit Prenatal Information Sheet

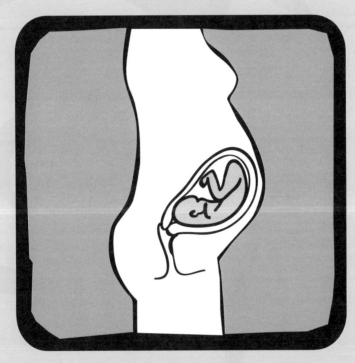

Goal: Monitor baby and your progress and learn to count fetal movements.

Prenatal Information Sheet: *28 Weeks Visit*

Goal: Monitor baby and your progress and learn to count fetal movements.

Today's visit

- **Every visit:** We will measure your uterine growth, blood pressure, weight, listen to your baby's heart rate, and discuss any concerns/questions you may have.
- Receive blood test for gestational diabetes.
- Check for pre-term labor.
- Review signs of pre-term and what to do if they occur.
- Learn how to do Fetal Movement Counts.
- You will have an additional blood test before receiving RhoGAM® (D-immunoglobulin) shot, if Rh negative.
- Register for Breast-feeding class, Childbirth classes and Labor & Delivery tour.

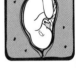

Today's visit

Your baby's growth

- Your baby's weight has doubled since your last visit! Your baby weighs about 2.5 lbs and is 10 inches long.
- The baby starts to lose the lanugo (fine hair), especially from the face. The baby has a large amount of cheesy-like substance (vernix) covering the body that protects the skin while the baby is living in the amniotic fluid. This vernix decreases on the skin as the baby grows.
- Your baby's eyebrows and eyelashes may be present now.
- The brain tissue also increases during this time.
- Now that you are 28 weeks, you should be feeling your baby move (kicks, rolls, twists, turns, and jabs) on a regular basis.

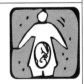

Your baby's growth

Your body's changes

- You've probably gained about 17 pounds.
- You may also start experiencing some swelling, and/or numbness or pain in your hands and wrists. Avoid sleeping on your hands or bending your wrists for long periods of time.

Your body's changes

Your family's changes

- Everyone needs help with child care options whether on a full, part time, or occasional basis.
- Active duty moms must list their child care providers upon return to work.
- Now is the time to explore the various child care options in your community.

Your family's changes

Signs to report **Signs to report immediately**
immediately

- Bright red vaginal bleeding, gush of fluid from the vagina, and/or four or more painful cramping contractions within an hour (after resting and emptying bladder).
- Persistent severe headaches, severe nausea, and vomiting.
- Fever over 100.5° F or 38° C.
- Visual changes such as bright white spots or loss of sight.
- Excessive thirst.
- Decrease in fetal movement (below ten movements/two hours).
- When in doubt, call your clinic, health care provider, or Labor & Delivery!

Notes:	Discussion:	Key points:

My BP:

_____

Your blood pressure

- Remember to report symptoms such as headache, blurred vision, sudden weight gain, swelling of hands and face, and decreased urination.

Your blood pressure

My weight:

_____

Your weight

- Try and eat a variety of foods.
- As a minimum you should eat these every day:
  - 6-11 servings of bread, cereal, rice or pasta
  - 3-5 servings of vegetables
  - 2-4 servings of fruit
  - 2-3 servings of protein such as poultry, fish, dry beans, meat, eggs & nuts
  - 3-5 servings of dairy products such as milk, yogurt, and cheese
- If needed, extra nutrients such as iron, vitamins B-6 and B-12, and calcium may be prescribed.

Your weight

Reference:
Prenatal
Fitness and
Exercise

Your exercise routine

- Now that your uterus is getting larger, you need to avoid exercises that require a lot of balance.
- Make sure you replace the energy burned during exercise with extra calories. These calories need to be nutritious for both you and your baby.

Your exercise

Consider breast-feeding

- Classes on breast-feeding will:
  - Help answer many questions.
  - Give you confidence in your ability to breast-feed.
  - Introduce you to other breast-feeding moms.
  - Reassure you that what you are doing is best for both you and your baby.

Consider breast-feeding

Fetal heart rate:

_____

Fetal heart rate

- This measurement will be done at each visit to monitor your baby's well-being.

Fetal heart rate

Fundal height

Fundal height

- The top of your uterus measures about 28 cm from your pubic bone.

Fundal height:

_____

Fetal Movement Count

Fetal Movement Count

- One very reassuring way to determine the baby's overall health and wellness is to record your baby's movements daily.
- By now, you probably know when your baby is most active. This may be before or after a meal, early in the morning, or at night when you go to bed. Each baby is unique.
- You should count your baby's movements whenever he or she is most active. This count should occur about the same time each day. You will need to record the time it takes for your baby to move 10 times.
- You should be able to feel at least ten movements within two hours.
- If you do not get ten movements within two hours, you should call or go to Labor & Delivery immediately with your movement chart. Do not wait until the next day or next appointment.

Fetal
Movement
Count:

_____

Pre-term labor guidelines

Pre-term labor guidelines (If you have any of the following symptoms you should follow the pre-term labor guidelines as listed in week 24.)

- **Report to your health care provider any of the following symptoms:**

  – Low, dull backache
  – Four or more uterine contractions per hour. Uterine contractions may be perceived by you as:
    - Menstrual cramps
    - Sensation of the "baby rolling up in a ball"
    - Abdominal cramping (may be associated with diarrhea)
    - Increased uterine activity compared to previous patterns
  – Increased pelvic pressure (may be with thigh cramps)

Notes:	Discussion:	Key points:

Pre-term labor guidelines (cont.)

- Sensation that "something feels different" (e.g., agitation, flu-like syndrome, and sensation that baby has "dropped").

• **You should report immediately:**

- Change in vaginal discharge such as change in color of mucus, leaking of clear fluid, spotting or bleeding, or a vaginal discharge with a fish-like odor

Pre-term labor
guidelines (cont.)

Gestational Diabetes (GD) testing

- High blood sugar puts your baby at risk for complications.
- High blood sugar usually develops towards the middle of your pregnancy.
- Risk factors include: being over age 25, overweight, family history of diabetes, ethnic background (Hispanic, African American, Native American, Asian), previous delivery of a baby over nine pounds.
- This test will determine if you have a normal response to a sugar load (glucola).
- If your blood sugar levels are high, further testing will be ordered.
- Often this condition can be controlled through special diet.

Gestational
Diabetes (GD)
testing

Resource: The Rh Factor: How It Can Affect Your Pregnancy (ACOG Pamphlet AP 027)

Rh (D) negative (Anti-D) prophylaxis

- Earlier in your pregnancy, you had a test to tell what your Rh (D) status was.
- Rh (D) negative women will have an additional blood test (antibody screen) and will usually receive RhoGAM® (D-Immunoglobulin) at this appointment.
- This shot will be repeated after delivery if baby has Rh (D) positive blood.

Rh (D) negative
(Anti-D)
prophylaxis

Summary of visit

Date of next visit: _____

Date for lab work/other medical tests:

_____

Summary of visit

Key points:	Discussion:	Notes:
Your next visit	**Your next visit** • **Every visit:** We will measure your uterine growth, blood pressure, weight, listen to your baby's heart rate, review fetal movement record, and discuss any concerns/questions you may have. • Sign up for classes (if not done already). • Receive domestic abuse screening. • Review pre-term labor signs.	
Questions for next visit	**Questions for next visit** ❑ _____ ❑ _____ ❑ _____ ❑ _____ ❑ _____	

Further information on the topics covered in this visit can be found at the end of the notebook.

Listing of medications/drugs does not represent endorsement by VA/DoD

32 Weeks Visit Prenatal Information Sheet

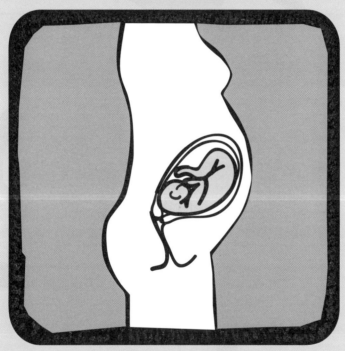

Goal: Prepare for your baby's arrival.

Prenatal Information Sheet: *32 Weeks Visit*

Goal: Prepare for your baby's arrival.

Today's visit

- **Every visit:** We will measure your uterine growth, blood pressure, weight, listen to your baby's heart rate, review the fetal movement record, and discuss any concerns/questions you may have.
- Check for pre-term labor.
- Receive domestic abuse screening.
- Sign up for classes such as Breast-feeding, Childbirth, Labor and Delivery, Postpartum and Newborn tour if not done yet.

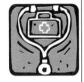

Today's visit

Your baby's growth

- Your baby weighs almost 4 pounds, and the length is 18-19 inches!
- Organ systems are now adequately developed.
- Most likely, your baby is in the "head down" position so you may feel most of his/her kicks and jabs under your ribs, or even a forceful blow to the cervix.

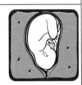

Your baby's growth

Your body's changes

- The top of your uterus is about 4-5 inches above your belly button by now.
- You may also notice that your back and pelvic area may feel different. The bones in your pelvis are moving and shifting to make room for the baby's head to pass through.
- As this happens, the ligaments around the pelvis also stretch, which can cause some discomfort in the hip joints, back, and front of the pelvis.

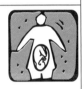

Your body's changes

Your family's changes

- You and your partner may become more anxious as the "big day" approaches.
- You may become more irritable and find that this can put a strain on your relationship.
- You'll probably find that it is harder to do all the things that you are used to doing, such as sleeping and moving quickly.
- Make sure you have a plan for getting to the hospital no matter when you need to go! This plan needs to include transportation, child and pet care options, and phone numbers.

Your family's changes

Signs to report immediately

- Bright red vaginal bleeding, gush of fluid from the vagina, and/or four or more painful cramping contractions within an hour (after resting and emptying bladder).
- Persistent severe headaches, severe nausea, and vomiting.
- Fever over 100.5° F or 38° C.
- Visual changes such as bright white spots or loss of sight.
- Excessive thirst.
- Decrease in fetal movement (below ten movements/two hours).
- When in doubt, call your clinic, health care provider, or Labor & Delivery!

Notes:	Discussion:	Key points:
My BP: _____	**Your blood pressure** • Remember to report symptoms such as headache, blurred vision, sudden weight gain, swelling of hands and face, and decreased urination.	Your blood pressure
My weight: _____	**Your weight** • Pregnancy increases your requirements for iron, calcium, folate, protein, and water. • Make sure to read food labels carefully. • Try to limit your refined sugars (honey, maple syrup, white, and brown sugars) by substituting with fruit and fruit juice concentrates.	Your weight
Reference: Prenatal Fitness and Exercise	**Your exercise routine** • You can continue to exercise right up to delivery and this may even help the delivery go more easily. • Don't exercise on an empty stomach and make sure you replace any fluids lost during exercise. • Avoid exercising in very hot and/or humid weather. • You may need to modify the intensity of your exercise routine according to your symptoms. Now is **not** the time to exercise to exhaustion or fatigue.	Your exercise
	Consider breast-feeding • The American Academy of Pediatrics, the American Academy of Family Practice and many other professional organizations recommend breast-feeding for the first 12 months, but any amount of breast-feeding is beneficial to your baby. • If you have any doubts or concerns about breast-feeding, let your provider know. We have many excellent resources to help you feel more comfortable and confident with breast-feeding.	Consider breast-feeding

Key points:	Discussion:	Notes:
Fetal heart rate	**Fetal heart rate** • This measurement will be done at each visit to monitor your baby's well-being.	Fetal heart rate: _____
Fundal height	**Fundal height** • The top of your uterus is 32 cm above your pubic bone or 4-5 inches above your belly button.	Fundal height: _____
Fetal Movement Count	**Fetal Movement Count** • Review fetal movement count record.	Fetal Movement Count: _____
Domestic abuse screen	**Domestic abuse screen** • Let your health care provider know if: – Within the last year, or since you have been pregnant, you have been hit, slapped, kicked, otherwise physically hurt, or forced to have sexual activities. • National Domestic Abuse Hotline: 1-800-799-7233	

Preparing for baby's arrival

- Most women go through the "nesting" phase a week or two before delivery.

- You'll probably clean everything in sight, so take it as a blessing in disguise.

- Plan, cook, and freeze some meals ahead of time. Keep a stock of basic staples, so you won't have to go to the store for basic food items.

- If friends offer to help, suggest that they cook a meal or two for you and your family.

- Baby's living area: Whether the baby has his or her own room, or is sharing a room with a sibling or with you, be sure that the area is clean and safe. Wash your baby's new sheets, blankets, and clothes in a mild detergent (or, if your machine has this feature, run them through an extra rinse) before you bring the baby home.

- After the baby comes home, you will have many new duties, a lot less sleep, and a lot less energy. So, our best advice, plan ahead.

Preparing for baby's arrival

Pre-term labor guidelines (*If you have any of the following symptoms you should follow the pre-term labor guidelines as listed in week 24.*)

- **Report to your health care provider any of the following symptoms:**

  – Low, dull backache

  – Four or more uterine contractions per hour. Uterine contractions may be perceived by you as:

    ■ Menstrual cramps

    ■ Sensation of the "baby rolling up in a ball"

    ■ Abdominal cramping (may be associated with diarrhea)

    ■ Increased uterine activity compared to previous patterns

  – Increased pelvic pressure (may be with thigh cramps)

  – Sensation that "something feels different" (e.g., agitation, flu-like syndrome, and sensation that baby has "dropped").

Pre-term labor guidelines

continued on next page

Key points:	Discussion:	Notes:
Pre-term labor guidelines (cont.)	**Pre-term labor guidelines (cont.)** • **You should report immediately:** – Change in vaginal discharge such as change in color of mucus, leaking of clear fluid, spotting or bleeding, or a vaginal discharge with a fish-like odor	
Summary of visit	**Summary of visit** Date of next visit: _____ Date for lab work/other medical tests: _____	
Your next visit	**Your next visit** • **Every visit:** We will measure your uterine growth, blood pressure, weight, listen to the baby's heart rate, review the fetal movement record, and discuss concerns/questions you may have. • Discuss your birth plan. • Have Group B Streptococcus (GBS) test.	
Questions for next visit	**Questions for next visit** ❑ _____ ❑ _____ ❑ _____ ❑ _____ ❑ _____	

Further information on the topics covered in this visit can be found at the end of the notebook.

Listing of medications/drugs does not represent endorsement by VA/DoD

36 Weeks Visit
Prenatal Information
Sheet

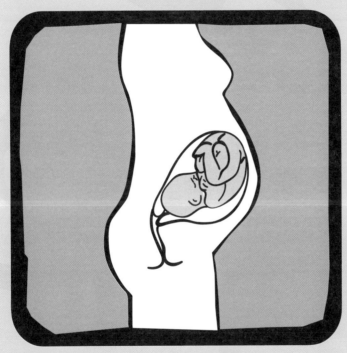

Goal: Begin preparations for your hospital experience.

Prenatal Information Sheet: *36 Weeks Visit*

Goal: Begin preparations for your hospital experience.

Today's visit

- **Every visit:** We will measure your uterine growth, blood pressure, weight, listen to baby's heart rate, review the fetal movement record, assess baby's position, and discuss any concerns/questions you may have.

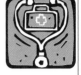

Today's visit

- Have test for Group B Streptococcus (GBS).
- Check for pre-term labor.
- Discuss birth plan.
- Complete necessary forms from your health care provider and take them to the Admissions Office for admission.

Your baby's growth

- Your baby probably weighs around 6 pounds now and is about 20 inches in length.
- Most likely, your baby is in the "head down" position. However, some babies settle into the head down position only a few days before delivery. If baby is in the breech (or butt down) position, your provider will discuss options to turn the baby to head down position.

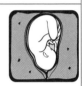

Your baby's growth

Your body's changes

- Easier breathing after the baby "drops" or moves down into pelvis. Some babies don't drop until after labor begins.
- More frequent urination after the baby "drops" down.
- Increased backache and heaviness.
- Pelvic and buttock discomfort.
- Increased swelling of the ankles and feet, and occasionally the hands and face.
- More frequent and more intense Braxton-Hicks (non-painful) contractions.

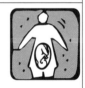

Your body's changes

Your family's changes

- More excitement and anxiety but also more impatience and restlessness as the delivery date nears are common.
- Apprehension about the baby's health and labor and delivery are common.
- Share these emotions.

Your family's changes

Signs to report immediately

Signs to report immediately

- Bright red vaginal bleeding, gush of fluid from the vagina, and/ or four or more painful cramping contractions within an hour (after resting and emptying bladder).
- Persistent severe headaches, severe nausea, and vomiting
- Fever over 100.5° F or 38° C.
- Visual changes such as bright white spots or loss of sight.
- Excessive thirst.
- Decrease in fetal movement (below ten movements/two hours).
- When in doubt, call your clinic, health care provider, or Labor & Delivery!

Notes:	Discussion:	Key points:

| My BP: | **Your blood pressure** | |
| | • Remember to report symptoms such as headache, blurred vision, sudden weight gain, swelling of hands and face, and decreased urination. | Your blood pressure |

My weight:	**Your weight**	
	• When making your choices from each food group, pick those that are low in fat and high in fiber and iron.	
	• With your enlarging uterus, you may need to eat smaller, more frequent meals.	Your weight

Reference: Prenatal Fitness and Exercise	**Your exercise routine**	
	• Regular exercise helps you keep fit during your pregnancy and feeling better during a time when your body is changing.	
	• Avoid overheating by drinking adequate amounts of fluids and wearing appropriate clothing.	Your exercise

| | **Consider breast-feeding** | |
| | • Breast milk is the ideal food for a baby and is easily digested. | Consider breast-feeding |

| Fetal heart rate: | **Fetal heart rate** | |
| | • This measurement will be done at each visit to monitor your baby's well-being. | Fetal heart rate |

| Fundal height: | **Fundal height** | |
| | • This measurement will be done at each visit to monitor the progress of your pregnancy. | Fundal height |

Key points:	Discussion:	Notes:
Fetal Movement Count	**Fetal Movement Count** • Review fetal movement count record.	Fetal Movement Count: _____
 **Fetal presentation**	**Fetal presentation** • The location of the baby's heartbeat in the lower half of your abdomen is a clue to your baby being in the head down position. • If the baby's position is not head-down, it can be confirmed by ultrasound. • Discussion of options includes performing an external version (turning the baby), planning for a vaginal delivery when possible, or scheduling a caesarean section.	
Group B Streptococcus	**Group B Streptococcus (GBS)** • GBS, bacteria commonly found in the vagina or rectum, can sometimes be passed on to the baby during labor and delivery. • Testing will determine if you have GBS. • Your provider will wipe the vaginal and rectal area and send the specimen to the lab. • Once completed, test results will be discussed with you at your next visit. • If the test is positive, you will receive antibiotics during labor.	Resource: Group B Streptococcus and Pregnancy (ACOG Pamphlet 105)
Birth plan	**Birth plan** • If you have a birth plan or any special requests, please let your nurse or health care provider know and we will do whatever we can to accommodate you and your family while also ensuring an optimal and healthy outcome.	

Preparing for baby's arrival

• Pack two bags, one for you and one for the baby. Your partner will have less to carry while helping you to Labor & Delivery.

Preparing for baby's arrival

• Bring things to make you comfortable: washcloths, extra socks, lip balm, hair items, basic toiletries. If you wear contact lenses, be sure to bring your case and a pair of glasses.

• Bring several pair of your oldest panties as you'll be bleeding quite a bit for a few days.

• If breast-feeding, be sure to bring a nursing bra or two.

• Feel free to bring your own nightgowns or pajama's, slippers, and robe, but we can also provide these items for your use while in the hospital.

• You will need clothes to go home in. Make sure they are comfortable, and, yes, you will still be wearing maternity clothes for awhile.

• For baby: bring an outfit to go home in, a blanket, and a car seat. You won't need these until the day of discharge.

• Feel free to bring a tape/CD player. Your tastes/preferences may change as you move through the different stages of labor, so you may want a variety of music options.

• Bring phone numbers of those you want to call immediately after the baby is born.

• Don't forget the camera! Bring extra film and batteries as back-up. You don't want to miss this! This is a once in a lifetime opportunity!

Pre-term labor guidelines

• **This is the last week you have to report pre-term labor symptoms. Remember you need to go into Labor & Delivery if you're having:**

Pre-term labor guidelines

    – More than 4 contractions per hour that do not ease up with drinking 3-4 glasses of water, emptying your bladder, and lying on your left side for an hour

    – Leaking of clear fluid, spotting or bleeding

    – Or other pre-term labor symptoms previously discussed.

Key points:	Discussion:	Notes:
Summary of visit	**Summary of visit** Date of next visit: _____ Date for lab work/other medical tests: _____	
Your next visit	**Your next visit** • **Every visit:** We will measure your uterine growth, blood pressure, weight, listen to your baby's heart rate, review the fetal movement record, assess baby's position, and discuss any concerns/questions you may have. • Discuss results of Group B Streptococcus (GBS) culture. • Have a vaginal exam to check for any changes in the cervix and strip your membranes if possible.	
Questions for next visit	**Questions for next visit** ☐ _____ ☐ _____ ☐ _____ ☐ _____ ☐ _____	

Further information on the topics covered in this visit can be found at the end of the notebook.

Listing of medications/drugs does not represent endorsement by VA/DoD

38–41 Weeks Visit Prenatal Information Sheet

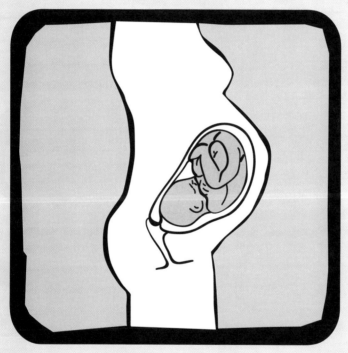

Goal: Preparing for the delivery and baby's arrival at home.

Prenatal Information Sheet: 38–41 Weeks Visit

Goal: Preparing for the delivery and baby's arrival at home.

Today's visit

Today's visit

- **Every visit:** We will measure your uterine growth, blood pressure, weight, listen to your baby's heart rate, review the fetal movement record, assess baby's position, and discuss any concerns/questions you may have.
- Vaginal exam: Your provider will check for any cervical opening or thinning and offer to strip membranes if possible.
- Sign up for any missed classes or tours.
- Discuss Group B Streptococcus (GBS) results.
- Update birth plan if needed.
- Make sure all necessary forms are completed and are at the Admissions Office.

Your baby's growth

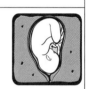

Your baby's growth

- Your baby probably weighs around 7 pounds now and is about 21 inches in total length.
- Most likely, your baby is in the "head down into the pelvis" position, but some babies won't drop into position until a few days before delivery or not until labor begins.
- You will be seen by a health care provider more frequently as your due date nears to ensure a safe delivery for both you and your baby.
- We know babies are usually mature enough to do very well on the outside beginning at 37 weeks. We also know babies continue to grow well within mom as long as everything is functioning normally. This functioning is what we will be watching closely with additional fetal testing beginning at 41 weeks.
- Labor will usually be induced at the 42nd week. Going longer then 42 weeks will put baby at increased risk for complications. Keep in mind that a majority of pregnancies are anywhere from 37 to 42 weeks long.

Your body's changes

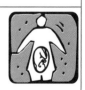

Your body's changes

- While baby's type of movement may change as he or she takes up more room in the uterus, it is still important to count and report any decrease in number of movements.
- Baby is getting big and you are getting tired. Avoid over-exhaustion; take frequent breaks and prop your feet up.
- If you have trouble sleeping, try a warm bath before bed, a soothing massage, pillows between your legs, or sleeping on your side.

Your family's changes

Your family's changes

- Keep in mind that you can deliver anytime from today till 42 weeks of pregnancy and that few babies are born on their due date.
- You and your family may become more frightened and/or frustrated if you have not delivered. Tips on conquering these fears and frustrations include:
  - Talking them over with your partner, friends, or health care provider.
  - Using relaxation techniques such as deep breathing, music, quiet walks, afternoon naps, and quiet time alone.
- Enjoy this time together and try to rest up for the big event.
- Review your labor and delivery coping techniques with your support person.

Signs to report immediately

Signs to report immediately

- Bright red vaginal bleeding, gush of fluid from the vagina, and/or four or more painful cramping contractions within an hour (after resting and emptying bladder).
- Persistent severe headaches, severe nausea, and vomiting.
- Fever over 100.5° F or 38° C.
- Visual changes such as bright white spots or loss of sight.
- Excessive thirst.
- Decrease in fetal movement (below ten movements/two hours).
- When in doubt, call your clinic, health care provider, or Labor & Delivery!

Notes:	Discussion:	Key points:
My BP: _____	**Your blood pressure** • It is still important to report to your health care provider any severe headache, blurring of vision, sudden weight gain, rapid swelling of hands and face, and decreased urination.	**Your blood pressure**
My weight: _____	**Your weight** • Total weight gain should be about 25 pounds unless you are over or underweight. Your weight gain is not all fat. It is mostly water in your body and the weight of the growing baby. • Weight gain generally slows down or ceases towards the end of your pregnancy.	**Your weight**
Reference: Prenatal Fitness and Exercise	**Your exercise routine** • Continue your exercises but modify intensity to avoid fatigue. • Don't forget to finish your exercise with an adequate cool down and relaxation period.	**Your exercise**
	Consider breast-feeding • Breast-feeding is not for every mother. Your decision will depend on life-style, desire, time and support. • Breast-feeding for even a few weeks has health benefits for the baby and mom. • You will need an extra 200 calories a day to produce milk for your baby.	**Consider breast-feeding**
Fetal heart rate: _____	**Fetal heart rate** • This measurement will be done at each visit to monitor your baby's well-being.	**Fetal heart rate**
Fundal height: _____	**Fundal height** • Measure uterine growth, and check to see if baby is dropping into the pelvis. You may feel this 'drop' as an increase in frequency of urination and easier breathing.	**Fundal height**

Key points:	Discussion:	Notes:

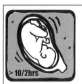

Fetal Movement Count

Fetal Movement Count

- Review Fetal Movement Count record.

Fetal Movement Count:

_____

Weekly cervical stripping

Weekly cervical stripping

- Towards the end of pregnancy, the cervix will start to prepare itself for going into labor. This preparation or "ripening" results in cervical softening (effacement) and opening (dilatation). The part of the membranes that was over the cervical opening can now usually be felt by a vaginal exam.
- In order to help prepare the cervix to go into labor and prevent your pregnancy from going much beyond your due date, your cervix may be "stripped".
- Your cervix is "stripped" by inserting a gloved finger between the membranes and the inner wall of the cervix. The finger is then swept in a circular motion around the inner cervix to separate the membranes from the cervical wall.
- Some women will get some contractions and some vaginal spotting as a result of this procedure. Some (but not many) will actually go into labor!

Postdate pregnancy plan

Postdate pregnancy plan

- If you have not delivered by 41 weeks, you will begin a "postdate pregnancy plan."
- This plan will include:
  – Non-stress tests twice a week
  – Weekly ultrasound measurement of amniotic fluid levels
  – Continued daily fetal movement recording
  – Continued weekly clinic visits
  – Possible induction at 42 weeks

Reference: What to Expect After Your Due Date (ACOG Pamphlet 069)

When you are admitted

When you are admitted

- Hopefully, by now, you have seen the Labor & Delivery area, are pre-admitted and have transportation and child/pet care arranged.

- Expect to be a little nervous. The big event is about to happen!

- Prior to admission, you will probably be given a vaginal exam to determine where you are in labor and both you and your baby's vital signs will be taken.

- If you are in active labor or your bag of water broke or you need close observation, you will be admitted and taken to a labor room where your baby's heart rate and your contractions will be monitored by an external fetal monitor (same monitor as used for the non-stress test you may have had). You will have your blood drawn and possibly an IV started at this time.

- Now you and your partner get to put all that practice to work! Remember each contraction only lasts less than 90 seconds and puts you one contraction closer to holding your baby.

- If you have any special requests, such as having the father cut the cord, or you want to breast feed immediately after delivery, let the staff know now. Don't forget the camera for your baby's very first pictures.

- Your placenta will deliver within 30 minutes after the baby is born but you are usually too occupied with baby to take much notice.

- This is a good time to put your baby to breast. This serves two functions: helps you bond with your new baby and decreases your blood loss by contracting your uterus.

Postpartum (after the delivery)

Postpartum (after the delivery)

- Even though you have usually worked hard and long to bring about this birth, most mothers are too excited to sleep. Enjoy this time. It is precious!

- The staff will be checking on both you and your baby frequently during this postpartum period. These checks are done to ensure both of you are doing well.

- If your child is male, you will need to decide on whether to have him circumcised. This procedure is usually done prior to hospital discharge. While there may be potential health benefits, at present, there is not enough medical evidence to recommend routine circumcision. Circumcision is a personal decision based on cultural, health, and religious beliefs.

- If you are having any problems caring for your newborn, let the staff know immediately. They are there to help you feel more comfortable and secure in your new role.

- The nursing staff will go over the basics of self and infant care. Ask questions and make sure you understand the information you are given.

Going home

Going home

- At the time of discharge, you will be given appointments for your baby's 2-week newborn check-up.

- Ask how to schedule your own 6-8 week postpartum appointment.

- Before leaving the hospital, your car seat will be evaluated and instructions given. The safest place for a newborn car seat is in the middle of the back seat facing the rear.

- If you need birth control, make sure it is obtained before leaving the hospital.

Post delivery appointments

- At the baby's appointment, your baby will be measured, weighed, and receive a complete physical exam.

- Parenting concerns such as feeding, bowel movements, sleep, and number of wet diapers will be discussed.

Post delivery appointments

- Be sure to write down questions you have and bring them with you to this visit.

- At your 6-8 week postpartum checkup, a pelvic examination will be done to see if your uterus has returned to normal along with a pap smear to check for cervical cancer.

- Your newborn is usually welcomed to accompany you to this visit. Check with your clinic and if you are bringing your baby, make sure you have a carriage or car seat for your baby during the exam.

- Your birth control method will be reviewed and revised as needed.

- If you, your baby, or your family are having problems adjusting, be sure to let your health care provider know.

Additional signs to report

- **Prior to your six week check-up, call your health care provider if you experience:**

  – Fever greater than 100.5° F or 38° C

  – Burning on urination

Additional signs to report

  – Increased pain near your vagina or surgical site

  – Foul smelling vaginal discharge

  – Swollen, painful, hot, red area on your leg

  – Extended periods of hopelessness or depression (more than 2-3 days a week)

Your next visit

- **Every visit:** We will measure your uterine growth, blood pressure, weight, listen to fetal heart rate, review fetal movement record, assess baby's position, and discuss any concerns/questions you may have.

Your next visit

- Discuss Postdate Pregnancy Plan if you have not delivered by 41 weeks.
- Schedule for twice a week Non-Stress Tests and weekly, ultrasound-amniotic fluid measurements beginning at your 41st week.
- Schedule weekly prenatal visits.

Questions for next visit

❑ _____

❑ _____

Questions for next visit

❑ _____

❑ _____

❑ _____

Further information on the topics covered in this visit can be found at the end of the notebook.

Prenatal Information Sheet Resources

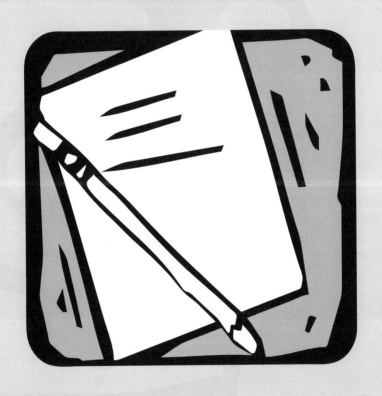

SAMPLE	**MEDICAL RECORD - CONSENT FORM** **Cystic Fibrosis Carrier Test**	

I understand that I am being asked to decide whether or not to have the Cystic Fibrosis test. This test can identify someone who is a carrier of this disease. By signing below, I show that I have been told what this test can and cannot do and that my questions were answered to my satisfaction.

By signing below I understand that:

1. This test can tell if I am a carrier of Cystic Fibrosis (CF), which means I have the gene but not the disease.
2. The risk of being a CF carrier depends on my race and ethnic background. For example,
   a. For European Caucasian, Ashkenazi Jewish couples
      (1) There is a 1 in 25 chance that one parent is a carrier.
      (2) There is a 1 in 625 chance that both parents are carriers.
   b. For Hispanic American couples
      (1) There is a 1 in 46 chance that one parent is a carrier.
      (2) There is a 1 in 2,116 chance that both parents are carriers.
   c. For African American couples
      (1) There is a 1 in 65 chance that one parent is a carrier.
      (2) There is a 1 in 4,225 chance that both parents are carriers.
   d. For Asian American couples
      (1) There is a 1 in 80 chance that one parent is a carrier.
      (2) There is a 1 in 8,100 chance that both parents are carriers.
3. I am the one to decide whether or not I am tested.
4. The test is not perfect. Some carriers are missed by the test.
5. If I am a carrier, in order to have a better idea of my baby's chances of getting the disease, testing the baby's father is needed.
6. If both parents are carriers, my baby has 1 in 4 chance of having CF. In that case, I will have the chance to have more testing to tell whether my baby has the disease.
7. Some parents may not wish to continue a pregnancy if they know their baby has CF.
8. Some individuals have not been able to get insurance because of the test results. I understand that my military health coverage will not be changed.
9. CF testing, like any DNA testing, can show that someone is not the real father. If the person who thought to be the father has a negative test, but the baby turns out to have the disease after birth, then it would be suspected that the real father is someone else. Possibly, other unknown family information may be uncovered.

I have read and understand the information provided to me about Cystic Fibrosis and have had my questions answered to my complete satisfaction.

I (circle one) **would** or **would not** like to have Cystic Fibrosis Carrier test.

Patient: _____
                (Print Name)

_____   _____
        (Signature)   (Date)

Witness: _____
                (Print Name)

_____   _____
        (Signature)   (Date)

SAMPLE	**MEDICAL RECORD - CONSENT FORM** Human Immunodeficiency Virus (HIV) Test	

I understand that I am being asked to decide whether or not to have the HIV test. This test is done to see if I have the HIV virus which causes Acquired Immunodeficiency Syndrome (AIDS). By signing below, I show that I have been told what this test can and cannot do and that my questions were answered to my satisfaction.

By signing below I understand that:

1. The HIV test detects antibodies to the Human Immunodeficiency Virus, which causes AIDS.

2. The HIV test is not 100% accurate. It can be falsely positive, meaning the test is positive when there is really no infection. Also, it can be falsely negative, meaning the test is negative when there really is an infection.

3. If I test positive, further testing is required.

4. If my test is truly positive, this does not mean that I have AIDS or will develop AIDS. However, it does mean that I can give the virus to another person.

5. If I am diagnosed with HIV by this test, my treatment during pregnancy, labor and delivery, and treatment of my baby during the first 6 weeks of his or her life will be drastically decrease the chance of my baby developing AIDS.

6. The Department of Defense has directed that all Active Duty patients receive HIV testing as a part of routine screening. For civilians, the decision to be tested is encouraged by not required.

7. HIV test results have caused some individuals to be denied insurance coverage. I understand that my military coverage will not be changed.

I have read and understand the information provided to me about HIV and have had my questions answered to my complete satisfaction.

I (circle one) **would** or **would not** like to have HIV testing.

Patient: _____
              (Print Name)

_____   _____
           (Signature)   (Date)

Witness: _____
              (Print Name)

_____   _____
           (Signature)   (Date)

SAMPLE	**MEDICAL RECORD - CONSENT FORM** **Maternal Serum Analyte Screen**	

I understand that I am being asked to decide whether or not to have the Maternal Serum Analyte Screen. The Maternal Serum Analyte Screen tests the mother's blood for substances made by the baby and the placenta. The amount of these substances in the blood, plus the maternal age are used to calculate the risk of certain problems with the baby including open neural tube defects, Down's syndrome (Trisomy 21), and Edwards syndrome (Trisomy 18). By signing below, I show that I have been told what this test can and cannot do and that my questions were answered to my satisfaction.

By signing below I understand that:

1. This is a screening test only: It DOES NOT provide a diagnosis; rather, it predicts the chance of a problem occurring.
2. The Maternal Serum Analyte Screen tests for an increased risk of a baby with certain birth defects such as an open neural tube birth defects, Down's syndrome, Edwards syndrome, and other related birth defects.
3. The Maternal Serum Analyte Screen, is not 100% accurate and is often abnormal when, in fact, the developing baby does not have one of these birth defects.
4. Open neural tube defects are abnormalities of the spinal cord or brain and occur in 1 or 2 out of every 1000 births. Overall, if I have an abnormal result on the Maternal Serum Analyte Screen, my baby has only a 4–7% risk of open neural tube defects.
5. Babies with Down's syndrome have a distinct physical appearance, mental retardation, and are at increased risk for other birth defects. About 1 in 800 babies are born with Down's syndrome (Trisomy 21), and the risk increases with the age of the mother. Overall, in women with an abnormal test result, the baby has a less than 3% risk of having Down's syndrome.
6. Babies with Edwards syndrome (Trisomy 18) have serious mental and physical disabilities. Only 1 out of 10 affected babies live past their first year. Only 1 in 8000 babies are born with Edwards syndrome and the risk increases with the age of the mother.
7. I am the one to decide whether or not I am tested.
8. As noted above, the test is not perfect. Some defects are missed and there are many abnormal Maternal Serum Analyte Screen results that turn out to have no association with birth defects. If there are abnormal results, I will need further testing to determine if anything is wrong with my baby.

I have read and understand the information provided to me about Maternal Serum Analyte Screen and have had my questions answered to my complete satisfaction.

I (circle one) **would** or **would not** like to have the Maternal Serum Analyte Screen.

Patient: _____
               (Print Name)

_____   _____
      (Signature)   (Date)

Witness: _____
               (Print Name)

_____   _____
      (Signature)   (Date)

Active Duty Information - Army

Congratulations!

With this pregnancy, you will be facing extraordinary changes in your life. Unlike your civilian counterparts, you also have to manage the impact that your pregnancy and military life will have on each other. The following information is provided to help you, the active duty expectant mother/soldier, make key decisions and chart the best course for your pregnancy.

Maternity uniforms:

You will be provided two sets of maternity uniforms (BDUs or whites). At most posts, you will need to take a memorandum from your commander requesting the issue and a copy of your pregnancy profile showing your due date to the Central Issuing Facility (CIF) or the unit supply room. These uniforms will be turned in upon your return from convalescent leave. Check with your command to inquire about specifics.

Education:

You are encouraged to participate in childbirth education programs offered at your facility. Childbirth education may include birthing classes, infant care information, breast-feeding education, exercise during pregnancy, and tours of the birthing unit and postpartum areas. Visit your local Medical Treatment Facility (MTF) and see what they have to offer.

Pregnancy profile:

Upon confirmation of your pregnancy (by examination or a lab test), you will be provided a physical profile that is effective for the duration of the pregnancy. Activities that are acceptable during pregnancy are specifically noted in the profile and include: specific stretching, aerobic conditioning at own pace, lifting up to 15 lbs, wearing a helmet, and carrying a rifle.

Although you are exempt from regular physical training (PT) and testing during your pregnancy, you are encouraged to participate in a pregnancy PT program, if available. Currently there is no standardized Army-wide PT program for pregnant and postpartum soldiers. However, many installations do have programs available. Obtain your health care provider's approval for any proposed exercise.

Additional limitations:

In addition to the physical profile, there are additional limitations regarding pregnant soldiers outlined in the Office of the Surgeon General Memorandum, dated 23 May 2001, *Pregnancy and Postpartum Physical Profiles*:

1. Except under unusual circumstances, the soldier will not be reassigned to or from CONUS during pregnancy. She may be reassigned within CONUS. A physician must clear the soldier prior to any reassignment.

2. An occupational history will be taken at the first visit to assess potential exposures in the soldier's work area. An occupational medicine physician or nurse usually performs this task. Listed are specific occupational concerns/limitations:

   a. No duty where nausea, easy fatigue, or sudden light-headedness would be hazardous to the soldier or others, to include aviation duty, Classes 1/1A/2/3, and work on ladders or scaffolding. The soldier may be granted permission to remain on flight status with approval by physician and Advanced Training Course supervisor.

   b. No duty with frequent or routine exposures to military fuels, (mogas, JP8, JP4) fuel vapors and/or handling.

   c. No indoor weapons training due to airborne lead concentrations and bore gas emissions.

   d. No work in motor pool where the soldier would be routinely exposed to potential hazards. This does not apply to pregnant soldiers who perform infrequent preventive maintenance checks and services (PMCS) on vehicles or to those pregnant soldiers who work in adequately ventilated areas adjacent to the motor pool (i.e., administrative offices).

   e. Avoid excessive vibrations, example: Driving in large (greater than 1¼ ton) ground vehicles on unpaved surfaces.

3. Exempt from all immunizations except influenza and tetanus-diphtheria.

4. Exempt from exposure to chemical and riot control agents, wearing load-bearing equipment to include web belt, and wearing MOPP gear at any time.

5. Duty:

   a. Can work shifts and continue to perform military duty until delivery. Soldiers with complicated pregnancies may have their duty modified by their health care provider.

   b. At 20 weeks of pregnancy:

      • Exempt from parade rest or standing at attention for longer than 15 minutes.

      • Exempt from swimming qualifications, drown proofing, field duty, and weapons training.

      • Exempt from riding in or driving vehicles larger than light medium tactical vehicles.

      • Exempt from all PMCS duties.

c. At 28 weeks of pregnancy, in addition to the above:

- 15 minute rest period allowed every 2 hours.
- Duty day not to exceed 8 hours. Workweek not to exceed 40 hours.
- Duty day begins with reporting for formation or duty and ends 8 hours later.

Convalescent leave:

Will be determined by attending physician following delivery. The usual time allotted is 42 days following a normal pregnancy and delivery. The physician also determines the amount of convalescent leave following other than a normal pregnancy and delivery (i.e. elective or spontaneous abortions, complications).

Postpartum profile:

Prior to leaving the hospital, your doctor will provide you with a postpartum profile. This temporary profile will be for 45 days beginning on the day of delivery and allows for PT at your own pace. Participation in a postpartum PT program is encouraged to assist you in returning to required fitness standards and transitioning back to unit PT.

Army Physical Fitness Test (APFT):

You are exempt from the APFT during pregnancy and for 180 days following delivery. At the end of 180 days, you will take a record APFT. Your unit may have you take diagnostic APFTs in preparation for the record test.

Family Care Plan:

Talk to your unit chain-of-command to insure that you have a family care plan in place taking the new addition to your family into consideration.

DEERS:

Soon after discharge from the hospital, you must stop by your personnel office or the nearest DEERS office to enroll your baby in DEERS. While at the Military Personnel Office (MILPO), take time to update your SGLI (Servicemembers' Group Life Insurance) and DD93 (Emergency Data Sheet).

TRICARE:

After enrolling in DEERS, you will be given the necessary forms for your baby's enrollment into TRICARE. Complete these forms and take to your nearest TRICARE office.

Finance:

Notify the Personnel Administration Center (PAC) of your new dependent.

Both parents active duty:

Both parents will need to update their SGLI and DD93. Only the sponsor needs to enroll the baby in DEERS, TRICARE, and notify PAC of new family member.

Congratulations again on the exciting road ahead of you. Hooah!

References:

Office of the Surgeon General Memorandum, dated 23 May 2001, *Pregnancy and Postpartum Physical Profiles*

http://chppm-www.apgea.army.mil/dhpw/Readiness/PPPT.aspx

Comment: Click last link for Current Pregnancy Profile Information

Site provides a succinct summary of the information contained in the specific references listed below.

AR 40-501 *Standards of Medical Fitness,* Pregnancy and Postpartum Profiles

AR 614-30 *Assignments, Details, and Transfers,* Overseas Service in Pregnancy

AR 600-8-10 *Leaves and Passes,* Postpartum Convalescent Leave

http://www.usapa.army.mil

Comment: Navigate through Official Documents, Army Administrative Publications

Site details considerations in pregnancy.

DOD Directive 1308.1 *DoD Physical Fitness and Body Fat Program*

http://www.dtic.mil/whs/directives/corres/html/13081.htm

Comment: Outlines postpartum exception to standard of fitness/body fat.

Active Duty Information - Navy/Marine Corps

Congratulations!

Expecting a baby is a wonderful, albeit daunting experience. And, of course, coordinating your life as a mother and as a member of the Navy/Marine Corps presents unique challenges. Your Navy health care team is ready to provide you with exceptional healthcare, as well as the information, education, and the support you will need, as you take this journey which will culminate in the delivery of a healthy infant and your healthy return to duty.

As you embark upon your journey and whether you deliver your baby at a Military Treatment Facility (MTF) or a civilian facility, please keep in mind that when a servicewoman receives confirmation of a pregnancy, she is responsible for notifying her commanding officer (CO) of her diagnosis within a designated timeframe. The health care provider will need to provide you with a completed Pregnancy Notification Form for use in notifying your CO. This Form will identify three time frames: Estimated Date of Confinement (EDC), the 20th week of pregnancy, and the 28th week of pregnancy. These dates are used by your command for planning purposes. The OPNAVINST 6000.1 and MCORDER 5000.12 Series provide guidance and detailed information regarding assignments and rest periods in relation to a servicewoman's pregnancy timeline. Navy and Marine Corps servicewomen are encouraged to consult their health care providers during the course of their pregnancy and recovery for guidance and support as they encounter work-related and healthcare issues that will require decision-making.

Useful policy references:

OPNAVINST 6000.1 Series: Guidelines Concerning Pregnant Servicewomen

MARINE CORPS ORDER 5000.12 Series: Marine Corps Policy on Pregnancy and Parenthood

MARINE CORPS ORDER P6100.12 Series: Marine Corps Physical Fitness Test and Body Composition Program Manual

OPNAVINST 6110.1 Series: Physical Readiness Program

OPNAVINST 1740.4 Series: U.S. Navy Family Care Policy

MARINE CORPS ORDER 1730.13 Series: Family Care Plans

NAVMEDCOMINST 6320.3 Series: Medical and Dental Care for Eligible Persons at Navy Medical Department Facilities

Internet references:

http://navymedicine.med.navy.mil/

http://www.hqmc.usmc.mil/hqmcmain.nsf/frontpage

http://www.bupers.navy.mil/

Active Duty Information - Air Force

Congratulations!

Whether you are pregnant for the first time or are an experienced mother, and whether your pregnancy was expected or a bit of a surprise, we want your pregnancy to be healthy, happy and successful. Pregnancy for anyone, let alone women on active duty in the military, can be a challenging experience. The Air Force has joined our sister services to create a plan of care, based on the best available current medical evidence, that will maximize your chances of a successful pregnancy. Our goal is to provide you with the care and education that you need to take home a healthy baby and be optimally prepared to care for your new addition. After all, your baby will be a new member to our Air Force family.

The plan of care and educational materials that are associated with these pregnancy guidelines as well as the requirements/limitations listed on your pregnancy profile will serve as a framework for your care during your pregnancy. There may be occasion to deviate from these guidelines due to your specific circumstances, potential pregnancy complications, local practices, and new medical information. Please remember that these are guidelines and are not a substitute for specific recommendations made by a qualified obstetrical health care provider.

At your first visit with your obstetrical health care provider, you should receive a document (pregnancy profile) that outlines some requirements and limitations regarding your activity during your pregnancy. As an Air Force service member, it is your responsibility to notify your supervisor regarding your pregnancy soon after pregnancy is diagnosed, and make sure that your supervisor gets a copy of the profile as soon as you receive it (AFI 48-123).

The pregnancy profile limits requirements for physical training, body weight requirements and environmental exposures. During your pregnancy and for at least six weeks following delivery, you are not worldwide qualified and must be removed from mobility status. Some of the limitations on your activity and military requirements extend as far as six months beyond your delivery. Although you are not required to perform formal physical training or weigh-ins, we strongly encourage you to eat a healthy diet and perform moderate exercise during your pregnancy. Most facilities offer programs on appropriate exercise, healthy diet, tobacco cessation, labor and delivery, and new moms classes and other programs, specifically for pregnant women. We encourage you to take advantage of these programs as well as some of the many other activities and resources that are available to you during your pregnancy.

We suggest you be cautious about information and advice you may receive from family members, friends, the internet or from other outside sources. While most of these sources are well-meaning and may provide important support, bad advice and inaccurate information is common. Please make sure to discuss your specific concerns with your health care provider.

Where possible, we encourage you to involve your baby's father or other important support person in your care. You are most likely to have a good outcome if you have a close, cooperative and positive interaction between you, your partner and your health care provider. Once again, congratulations. We look forward to serving you.

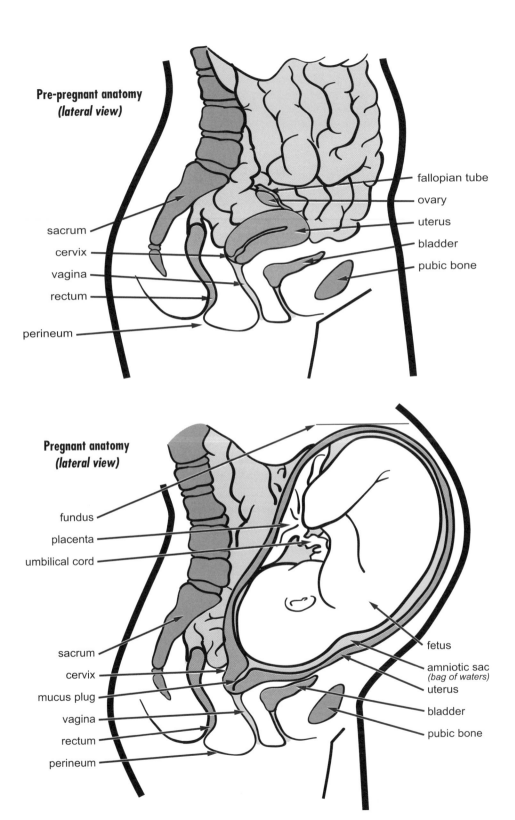

Pre-pregnant anatomy
(lateral view)

fallopian tube

ovary

uterus

sacrum

bladder

cervix

vagina

pubic bone

rectum

perineum

Pregnant anatomy
(lateral view)

fundus

placenta

umbilical cord

sacrum

cervix

fetus

mucus plug

amniotic sac
(bag of waters)

vagina

uterus

rectum

bladder

perineum

pubic bone

Common Discomforts & Annoyances of Pregnancy

All these discomforts/annoyances are a normal part of pregnancy and will end eventually. Try the hints given below. If you don't get relief, talk to your doctor, midwife or nurse about other possible measures to try.

Discomforts of Pregnancy

Discomfort	When	What you can do to help
Ankle/foot swelling	Second trimester till end	• Wear comfortable shoes or sandals and avoid high heels. • While sitting, prop your feet up (even a few inches up helps) and don't cross your legs. • Continue drinking lots of fluids.
Breast tenderness	Begins early and continues	• Wear a good support or athletic bra day and night. • Soak in a warm bath.
Breast leakage	Begins during the second trimester	• Wear breast pads that don't have any plastic linings. • Avoid harsh soaps, creams or ointments.
Bleeding gums	Throughout	• Use a very soft tooth brush and gently brush teeth. • Get routine dental care.
Constipation	Second trimester until the end	• Eat foods high in fiber (bran cereal, green leafy vegetables, whole grain breads, fruits) every day. • Drink lots of fluids to include: water, soups, milk, and fruit juices, especially prune juice. • Exercise each day. (Increased physical activity will help move food through your bowel.) • Walk after meals. • Avoid laxatives and enemas unless prescribed by your doctor or midwife.
Contractions (Braxton-Hicks)	After 20th week	• Lie down on your left side for about 20 minutes. • Drink two to three glasses of juice or water. • Walk around.

Table continued on next page.

Discomforts of Pregnancy

Discomfort	When	What you can do to help
Dizziness	As your uterus enlarges	• Get up from lying down slowly. • Do not go too long between meals and carry healthy snacks with you. • Drink lots of fluids. • If you get dizzy, lie down on your side or bend forward with your head down close to your knees.
Enlarging belly and breasts	Second half of pregnancy	• Sleep on your side with a pillow between your legs and lower abdomen. • Wear loose, comfortable clothing. • Wear a supportive bra even to bed.
Fatigue or tiredness	Early in pregnancy and again in the last month	• Take extra naps during the day if possible. • Continue exercise but not to the point of exhaustion. • Try to get at least 8 hours sleep a night.
Flatulence	Anytime, especially after 20 weeks	• Try to schedule your daily bowel movement. • Avoid gas-forming foods such as beans, cabbage and sodas. • Increase bulk and water to diet. • Increase exercise.
Food cravings	First half of pregnancy	• OK to indulge a bit as long as diet is otherwise healthy and food choice is not harmful.
Frequent urination	Begins early, gets better mid-pregnancy, then increases towards the end of pregnancy when baby drops.	• Know where the bathrooms are when out and about. • Don't cut back on fluids. • Expect to make many trips to the bathroom, day and night. • Avoid drinking lots of fluids before bedtime.

Table continued on next page.

Discomforts of Pregnancy

Discomfort	When	What you can do to help
Headaches	First half	• Avoid eyestrain. • Rest eyes frequently and take frequent computer breaks. • Use mild analgesics as directed. • Avoid aspirin and other pain medications, unless you have discussed their use with health care provider.
Heartburn	Second trimester till end	• Eat more frequent and small meals. • Eat slowly and chew your food well. • Avoid deep fried, greasy, and spicy foods. • Drink fluids between your meals. • Go for a walk after meals. • Avoid lying down right after eating. • Antacids, as directed, are safe and effective.
Hemorrhoids	Anytime	• Avoid constipation. • Apply cold witch hazel pads or hemorrhoid ointment. • Do your Kegel exercises. • Take sitz baths.
Increased perspiration	Anytime	• Increase fluids. • Wear easily washable, comfortable, loose fitting clothing. • Practice good hygiene.
Increased saliva	First trimester	• Gum and hard candy– watch excess calories • Use mouthwash. • Avoid starches.
Increased vaginal discharge	Throughout pregnancy	• Wear cotton underwear. Don't wear sanitary napkins or mini pads. • Avoid nylon panty hose, feminine hygiene soaps or sprays. • **DON'T douche.** • Inform your health care provider immediately, if your vaginal discharge is yellow or greenish, thick and cheesy, or has a strong fish-like odor, or if there is soreness, itching or burning.

Table continued on next page.

Discomforts of Pregnancy

Discomfort	When	What you can do to help
Leg cramps	Second half of pregnancy	• Extra potassium or calcium may help. Try eating a banana every day or drinking a glass of milk. • When you get a leg cramp: Stand up on flat surface or point your ankle and toes as if you were standing or try walking or curling your toes.
Ligament pain (sharp pulling sensation on either side of the lower abdomen)	Increases with increasing uterine size	• Support your weight with your hands when changing positions. • Move slower. • Mild analgesic may help. • Apply ice to affected side. • Use maternity girdle/belt. • Lean back in a slant position supporting your back with your knees bent.
Light headed & dizzy	Begins early and continues	• Stop what you are doing and lie on your left side with your legs up for short period of time. • Get up slowly from a lying down position.

Low backache	Second half of pregnancy	• Good body mechanics help:
		  – Keep your back straight and your head up.
		  – Avoid bending at the waist to lift things.
		  – Wear comfortable flat shoes– No high heels!
		  – Don't stretch to reach high places.
		  – Avoid prolonged standing.
		  – Keep one foot on a stool with leg bent.
		• Move about frequently.
		• Get back rubs.
		• Use a firm mattress or put a board under your mattress.
		• Do pelvic rock exercises to strengthen your back.

Table continued on next page.

Discomforts of Pregnancy

Discomfort	When	What you can do to help
Nasal stuffiness & bleeding	1st trimester and again at term	• Use humidifier/vaporizer if air is dry. • Can use over-the-counter (OTC) decongestant such as Pseudoephedrine as directed. • Use a saline nasal spray. • Avoid using nasal decongestant sprays. • If your nasal stuffiness occurs often and is difficult to control, tell your health care provider. • Blow your nose gently.
Nausea (Morning Sickness)	Occurs in early pregnancy and usually improves after first trimester.	• Nibble some crackers before getting up in the morning and when you are feeling queasy. • After getting up in the morning, wait an hour to drink any liquids. • Eat small snacks throughout the day instead of big meals. • Avoid any strong odors. • Drink liquids between meals rather than with meals. • Stay away from greasy, smelly, or spicy foods. • Chew gum and suck on hard candy. • Sip on room temperature ginger ale or clear sodas. • Sit and put your head down between your legs. • Talk to your health care provider if your symptoms continue.
Sleeplessness	Anytime but especially last trimester	• Try a warm bath prior to bed. • Do not have stimulating activity before bed. • Use relaxation techniques. • Get in a comfortable position to sleep; place pillows between legs and under lower abdomen.

Table continued on next page.

Discomforts of Pregnancy

Discomfort	When	What you can do to help
Varicose veins	Increases as pregnancy increases	• Put support hose, ace wraps or elastic stockings on in bed before lowering feet down. • Avoid tight clothing. • Avoid crossing legs. • Practice good posture.
Vision changes	Throughout pregnancy	• Don't buy a new prescription for your glasses as you will probably return to pre-pregnant vision after delivery. • Take frequent eye breaks. • May not be able to wear contact lenses during pregnancy.

References:
Florida State University Center for Prevention and Early Intervention (1999).
"Partners for a Healthy Baby: Home Visiting Curriculum for Expectant Families".
Cunningham, F.G., et al. (2001) Williams Obstetrics (21st ed.), McGraw-Hill.
Varney, H. (1997). Varney's Midwifery (3rd ed.). Jones and Bartlett.

Fetal Movement Counting Chart

Go to Labor and Delivery if less than 10 movements in 2 hours (120 minutes)

Date														
120 min.														
110 min.														
100 min.														
90 min.														
80 min.														
70 min.														
60 min.														
50 min.														
40 min.														
30 min.														
20 min.														
10 min.														
Start time														
Weeks pregnant														

Counting your baby's movements is an excellent way of knowing that your baby is doing well. It is also a great excuse for you to get off your feet, relax and get in touch with your baby. You should begin counting your baby's movements when he or she is usually most active and you have time to concentrate. Begin your count around the same time each day and start by lying down on your left side with hands over your uterus. Write the time you begin your counts on the chart in the "start time" row. Also write down the date in the top row marked 'date' and the number of weeks you are pregnant in the bottom row. Count 10 distinct movements and note how long it took, i.e. 15 minutes, two hours, whatever time it took. Put an "X" in the time box closest to the total time it took for your baby to move 10 times.

If you have not felt 10 movements in two hours you will need to be monitored in Labor & Delivery to make sure your baby is OK. You may want to call Labor & Delivery to tell them you are on your way (but don't let the phone call delay you from going in). In most cases your baby is just fine, but it is always better to be safe than sorry.

Bring this chart with you to your next visit and any time you go to Labor & Delivery.

Fetal Movement Counting Chart

Go to Labor and Delivery if less than 10 movements in 2 hours (120 minutes)

Date							
120 min.							
110 min.							
100 min.							
90 min.							
80 min.							
70 min.							
60 min.							
50 min.							
40 min.							
30 min.							
20 min.							
10 min.							
Start time							
Weeks pregnant							

Counting your baby's movements is an excellent way of knowing that your baby is doing well. It is also a great excuse for you to get off your feet, relax and get in touch with your baby. You should begin counting your baby's movements when he or she is usually most active and you have time to concentrate. Begin your count around the same time each day and start by lying down on your left side with your hands over your uterus. Write the time you begin your counts on the chart in the "start time" row. Also write down the date in the top row marked "date" and the number of weeks you are pregnant in the bottom row. Count 10 distinct movements and note how long it took, i.e. 15 minutes, two hours, whatever time it took. Put an "X" in the time box closest to the total time it took for your baby to move 10 times.

If you have not felt 10 movements in two hours you will need to be monitored in Labor & Delivery to make sure your baby is OK. You may want to call Labor & Delivery to tell them you are on your way (but don't let the phone call delay you from going in). In most cases your baby is just fine, but it is always better to be safe than sorry.

Bring this chart with you to your next visit and any time you go to Labor & Delivery.

Fetal Movement Counting Chart

Go to Labor and Delivery if less than 10 movements in 2 hours (120 minutes)

Date													
120 min.													
110 min.													
100 min.													
90 min.													
80 min.													
70 min.													
60 min.													
50 min.													
40 min.													
30 min.													
20 min.													
10 min.													
Start time													
Weeks pregnant													

Counting your baby's movements is an excellent way of knowing that your baby is doing well. It is also a great excuse for you to get off your feet, relax and get in touch with your baby. You should begin counting your baby's movements when he or she is usually most active and you have time to concentrate. Begin your count around the same time each day and start by lying down on your left side with hands over your uterus. Write the time you begin your counts on the chart in the "start time" row. Also write down the date in the top row marked 'date' and the number of weeks you are pregnant in the bottom row. Count 10 distinct movements and note how long it took, i.e. 15 minutes, two hours, whatever time it took. Put an "X" in the time box closest to the total time it took for your baby to move 10 times.

If you have not felt 10 movements in two hours you will need to be monitored in Labor & Delivery to make sure your baby is OK. You may want to call Labor & Delivery to tell them you are on your way (but don't let the phone call delay you from going in). In most cases your baby is just fine, but it is always better to be safe than sorry.

Bring this chart with you to your next visit and any time you go to Labor & Delivery.

Go to Labor and Delivery if less than 10 movements in 2 hours (120 minutes)

Date							
120 min.							
110 min.							
100 min.							
90 min.							
80 min.							
70 min.							
60 min.							
50 min.							
40 min.							
30 min.							
20 min.							
10 min.							
Start time							
Weeks pregnant							

Counting your baby's movements is an excellent way of knowing that your baby is doing well. It is also a great excuse for you to get off your feet, relax and get in touch with your baby. You should begin counting your baby's movements when he or she is usually most active and you have time to concentrate. Begin your count around the same time each day and start by lying down on your left side with hands over your uterus. Write the time you begin your counts on the chart in the "start time" row. Also write down the date in the top row marked 'date' and the number of weeks you are pregnant in the bottom row. Count 10 distinct movements and note how long it took, i.e. 15 minutes, two hours, whatever time it took. Put an "X" in the time box closest to the total time it took for your baby to move 10 times.

If you have not felt 10 movements in two hours you will need to be monitored in Labor & Delivery to make sure your baby is OK. You may want to call Labor & Delivery to tell them you are on your way (but don't let the phone call delay you from going in). In most cases your baby is just fine, but it is always better to be safe than sorry.

Bring this chart with you to your next visit and any time you go to Labor & Delivery.

Immunizations:

Immunizations offer protection against certain diseases and are usually given during our childhood. Some immunizations can be given during pregnancy while others cannot. You will be screened for several of the diseases that you (and your unborn baby) might be at risk for. This screening is through blood tests (Rubella, Hepatitis B) or through your childhood disease history (measles, mumps, chickenpox) or immunization history (tetanus). It is important to know if you are protected against these diseases, and, if not, what can be done to decrease your risk of getting a disease. If you are at risk for any of the diseases screened for, immunization will be offered during your pregnancy (if safe) or immediately after the baby is born. If you cannot avoid travel to foreign countries during your pregnancy, talk to your health care provider to see what can be done to lessen your risk from other diseases such as yellow fever and malaria.

Immunizations

Vaccine/ Disease	Screening for Immunity	Affects of Disease on baby	Use in Pregnancy
MMR: Measles, Mumps and Rubella- (German Measles)	Childhood disease history obtained at first visit. Rubella screened through a blood test at initial visit.	**Measles:** increased risk of miscarriage and may possibly cause birth defects **Mumps:** increased risk of first trimester miscarriage **Rubella:** Severe congenital defects especially when disease occurs early in pregnancy	Immunization is not safe during pregnancy. Avoid gatherings of young children and people with disease while pregnant. Receive immunization after delivery and use birth control for three months after delivery.
Influenza: Flu	None	Possible increase in miscarriages	Safe to use in pregnancy
Hepatitis B	Screened through a blood test at initial visit	Possible increase in miscarriage and pre-term birth, neonatal hepatitis infection	Safe to use in pregnancy for women at high risk of exposure such as laboratory personnel, etc.
Tetanus-diphtheria	Tetanus shot/booster required every 10 years.	60% fetal death	Safe in pregnancy

Table continued on next page.

Immunizations (cont.)

Vaccine/ Disease	Screening for Immunity	Affects of Disease on baby	Use in Pregnancy
Varicella (chicken pox)	Childhood disease history obtained at first visit.	Increased deaths during first few weeks of birth	Safe for women exposed to varicella during pregnancy
Smallpox	None	See www.vaccines.army.mil	Immunization is not safe for pregnant women and pregnancy should be avoided 4 weeks after getting the smallpox vaccine.
Anthrax	None	See www.vaccines.army.mil	As a precaution, pregnant women should not be routinely vaccinated with anthrax vaccine.

Cunningham, F.G., et al. (2001) Williams Obstetrics (21st ed.), McGraw-Hill. Varney, H. (1997). Varney's Midwifery (3rd ed.). Jones and Bartlett.

Nutrition in Pregnancy

What you eat effects your baby's development! Make healthier choices during pregnancy; you're nourishing a growing child. Do not drink alcohol and avoid tobacco use and second-hand smoke. Concentrate on taking in good foods like milk, fruits, and vegetables through a healthy diet.

A few basic pregnancy dietary rules to follow are:

1. Drink at least 8 glasses or 2 quarts of water each and every day.

2. Eat 6-7 ounces of meat each day. Avoid raw or under cooked fish (sushi), meat, poultry, eggs and hot dogs. Avoid swordfish, shark, king mackerel and tile fish.

   Examples of a serving of protein-rich foods include:

   - ½ chicken breast = 3 ounces of meat; 1 drumstick = 2 ounces

   - Any meat the size of a deck of playing cards = 3 ounces of meat

   - ½ cup all beans (exception: green beans) = 1 ounce of meat

   - 1 egg = 1 ounce of meat; 1 ounce of most nuts = 1 ounce of meat

3. At least half of your food intake should be carbohydrates. Avoid raw sprouts, unpasteurized juices, milk and soft cheeses such as brie, feta, and roquefort.

   Examples of high-quality carbohydrates include:

   - Fruits

   - Vegetables - Peas and beans are the best sources

   - Whole grains

   - Low-fat dairy products

4. Limit the amount of fat in your diet; a small amount is fine but don't overdo it.

   Examples of high quality fats include:

   - Liquid vegetable oils or olive oil in small amounts.

5. Make sure you are taking in adequate vitamins and minerals each day.

   Calcium: Required for fetal bone, teeth, nerves, heart and muscle development and prevention of osteoporosis later in life. Foods rich in calcium include: all dairy products, turnips, mustard greens and broccoli. Calcium-fortified products are also acceptable (i.e., orange juice, bread, some cereals). You need 1200 to 1500mg daily.

Folate: A B-vitamin shown to reduce birth defects of the spinal cord and brain. It is found in many fortified cereals, citrus fruits, organ meats and dried peas and beans. Try to eat washed vegetables raw. Keep your fresh fruits refrigerated. The folate found in vegetables is destroyed in cooking water, try steaming or stir-frying rather than boiling them. The folate content of dried beans and peas, however, is not destroyed with cooking. You need 0.6mg or 600 micrograms of folate a day.

Iron: The increased amount of iron your body requires is dependent on how much iron you have stored. You need 30mg of iron per day; your body absorbs animal sources best. To help absorb the iron you are eating, take in Vitamin-C (citrus fruits) at the same time. If you are not taking in the daily recommended vitamins and minerals, you should take vitamin supplements.

6. Limit caffeine to 2–3 servings per day.

7. Sugar substitutes should be used in moderation during pregnancy. Some caution should be exercised with the use of saccharin since saccharin can cross the placenta.

Remember what you eat does count. See the table, "Common Discomforts & Annoyances of Pregnancy" in the Resource Section of this booklet for tips on dealing with nausea, vomiting, heartburn, and constipation.

Food Guide Pyramid: A Guide to Healthier Eating

Fats, Oils, Sweets
Limit

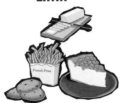

Milk Group
3–5 servings a day
Need 1200–1500mg
daily

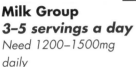

Protein Group
2–3 servings a day,

total of 6–7
ounces
daily

Vegetable Group
3–5 servings a day

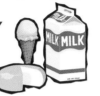

The best
sources of
fiber are potatoes with skin, carrots,
peas, broccoli, cauliflower, and corn.

Fruit Group
2–4 servings a day

The best sources
of fiber are
apples,
oranges, pears,
and strawberries.

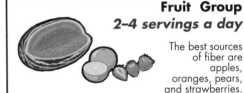

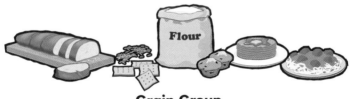

Grain Group
6–11 servings a day
The best sources of fiber are whole grains and breakfast cereals.

Avoid too much weight gain.

- Limit all juice to two 4-ounce servings per day or one 12-ounce regular soda.
- You're not "eating for two." At 4 months, add an extra 300 calories per day. Examples of 300 calories include a sandwich with two ounces of meat or a small peanut butter and jelly sandwich or two 8-ounce glasses of milk.
- A value meal at typical fast food restaurant has about 1500 calories, which is almost a full days worth of calories!
- Limit fried foods and high fat meats such as ribs and sausage. Choose lean cuts of meat such as "loin" cuts and trim visible fat.
- Use mayonnaise, salad dressings, and oils sparingly.
- If you need to, just cut back.
- Remember to exercise. Walking and being active in your daily routine counts!
- Make an appointment with a dietitian to address your individual needs.

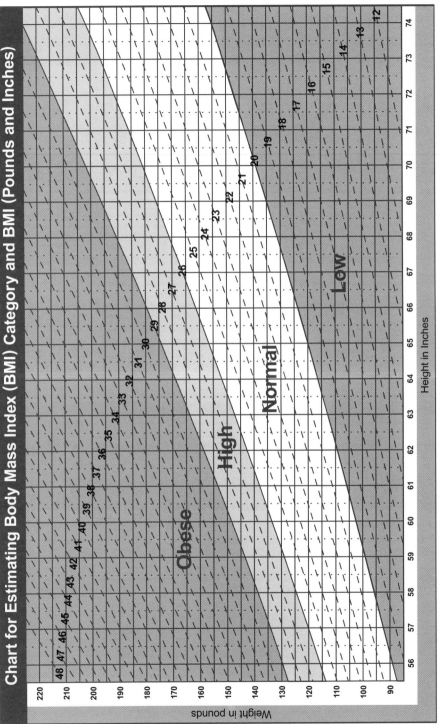

Chart for Estimating Body Mass Index (BMI) Category and BMI (Pounds and Inches)

Directions:

To find BMI category (e.g., obese), find the point where the woman's height and weight intersect. To estimate BMI, read the bold number on the dashed line that is closest to this point.

Reprinted with permission from *Nutrition During Pregnancy and Lactation, An Implementation Guide*. Copyright 1992 by the National Academy of Sciences, Courtesy of the National Academy Press, Washington, D.C.

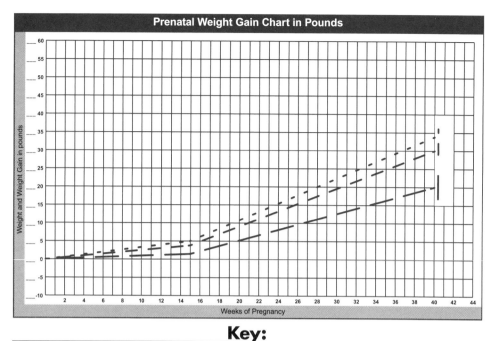

Prenatal Weight Gain Chart in Pounds

Weight and Weight Gain in pounds

Weeks of Pregnancy

Key:
Prepregnancy BMI < 19.8 (- - - - - - - -)
Pre-pregnancy BMI < 19.8–26.0 (normal body weight) (– – – – –)
Pre-pregnancy BMI > 26.0 (— — —)

Weight Record			
Date	Weeks of Gestation	Weight	Notes

Sexually Transmitted Diseases (STDs), Infections, & Pregnancy

Sexually transmitted diseases affect one in four Americans at some time in their life. During your pregnancy you will be tested for several of the STDs and treated if needed. Many of the STDs require that you and your partner be treated to avoid re-infection.

STDs can cause serious harm to your baby if left untreated. Most STDs can be treated during pregnancy, but treatment does not prevent you from becoming infected again or being infected with a new STD during this pregnancy. Using condoms and avoiding sexual contact with an infected person can help protect you against STDs. If, at anytime during your pregnancy, you think you have been exposed to an STD or have any symptoms of an STD (vaginal itching, odor, or abnormal discharge) let your health care provider know. You will be tested and treated.

This list is alphabetically arranged and includes some of the more common and more potentially harmful STDs. This does not cover all of them, as there are over twenty known STDs.

Chlamydia:

- **Possible effects on baby:** Baby has a 20-50% chance of becoming infected while passing through the birth canal resulting in pneumonia or an eye infection.

- **Signs and symptoms of infection:** More than 50% of all infections are without symptoms. You can experience burning on urination or unusual vaginal discharge.

- **Treatment:** Antibiotic pills for you. Antibiotic ointment to baby's eyes at birth.

- **Testing:** Cervical culture at the time of your initial pap smear.

Gonorrhea (Drip, clap, dose):

- **Possible effects on baby:** Baby can become infected as it passes through the birth canal. This infection can result in conjunctivitis (redness of the eye), blindness and/or a serious generalized infection.

- **Signs and symptoms of infection:** Burning on urination, unusual vaginal discharge or no symptoms at all.

- **Treatment:** Antibiotic pills for you and an antibiotic ointment for the baby's eyes at birth.

- **Testing:** Cervical culture at the time of your initial pap smear.

Genital warts:

- **Possible effects on baby:** Baby can get laryngeal papillomas (benign tumors on the vocal cords) from passing through an infected birth canal.

- **Signs and symptoms of infection:** Skin tags or warts that can be small or large, soft or hard, raised or flat, single, or in clusters like cauliflower.

- **Treatment:** Usually delay treatment until after delivery but may be removed in pregnancy if absolutely necessary. If large enough to block the birth canal, you may need a cesarean section.

- **Testing:** Let your health care provider know if you think you have warts.

Hepatitis B:

- **Possible effects on baby:** Can pass to your baby during the pregnancy resulting in liver damage and risk of death.

- **Signs and symptoms of infection:** You often have no symptoms. You can have yellowing of the skin and eyes, loss of appetite, nausea, vomiting, stomach and joint pain, or extreme tiredness.

- **Treatment:** Vaccine, immune globulin, and a baby bath after delivery can help protect baby from becoming infected.

- **Testing:** Blood test at initial visit.

Herpes Simplex Virus (Herpes):

- **Possible effects on baby:** Can be transmitted to baby during delivery if mother has blisters near term. Can cause severe disease and death of newborn but transmission is extremely rare, even with vaginal births.

- **Signs and symptoms of infection:** Fluid-filled sores in the genital area that may itch, burn, tingle or cause pain

- **Treatment:** If active infection occurs at or near your delivery date, you may need cesarean section within 4-6 hours of your bag of waters breaking.

- **Testing:** Tell your health care provider immediately if you think you have an outbreak (looks like warts). Cultures of the blisters can be done.

HIV (AIDS):

- **Possible effects on baby:** Can pass infection to baby while pregnant, during birth or through breast-feeding. Can cause serious complications and death to baby.

- **Signs and symptoms of infection:** Often times no symptoms of HIV.

- **Treatment:** Medication called AZT® can decrease transmission to baby.

- **Testing:** Blood test at initial visit.

Syphilis (Syph, pox, bad blood):

- **Possible effects on baby:** Miscarriage, stillbirth or damage to baby's bones, teeth and brain.

- **Signs and symptoms of infection:** Painless sores in genital area.

- **Treatment:** Antibiotics for the mother.

- **Testing:** Blood test at first visit.

Trichomonas (Trich):

- **Possible effects on baby:** May increase chance of pre-term labor.

- **Signs and symptoms of infection:** Common in pregnancy. You may have an increase in odorous, thin or thick, white, yellow-green/gray vaginal discharge with itching.

- **Treatment:** Flagyl® pills can be given safely after the first trimester.

- **Testing:** Tell your health care provider. Your vaginal discharge will be examined under a microscope.

Yeast (Candidiasis):

- **Possible effects on baby:** Baby can get a mouth infection (thrush) while passing through an infected birth canal

- **Signs and symptoms of infection:** Vaginal itching or burning pain, which increases with urination and sex. Can also occur without sexual transmission. More common in pregnancy.

- **Treatment:** Vaginal creams or suppositories. Nystatin® for baby.

- **Testing:** Let your health care provider know if you are experiencing any symptoms. A vaginal secretion sample will be looked at under the microscope.

References:
Partners for a Healthy Baby: Home Visiting Curriculum for Expectant Families 1999 Florida State University Center for Prevention and Early Intervention Policy Sexually Transmitted Diseases, WA State Department of Health, Office of SED Services, Oley, WAS DOH pub 347-002.

Listing of medications/drugs does not represent endorsement by VA/DoD

Testing & Monitoring During Pregnancy

At each of your goal-centered visits, your health care provider will be monitoring the health of you and your baby through a variety of techniques. These techniques include blood pressure checks, uterine growth measurements, your weight and detailed questioning of your activities, feelings and eating patterns. These assessments can reassure both you and your health care provider that you and your baby are doing well.

Another means of checking your baby's health is through a variety of fetal tests. One such test is the Fetal Movement Count. Beginning at 28 weeks, your health care provider will instruct you on how to count the baby's activity through fetal movement counts. As long as your baby's activity stays above the minimum ten movements in two hours or doesn't drastically decrease you can be assured that the baby is doing fine. Other tests such as Non-Stress Testing and measuring the amount of your amniotic fluid (bag of waters) by ultrasound are routinely begun on all women at 41 weeks. This is the time when the placenta is starting to age and may not be able to meet all the baby's needs. In addition, mother's tests such as Biophysical Profiles and Contraction Stress tests are used if more information is needed in certain situations due to either mom's or baby's health.

Fetal testing includes:

- Ultrasound exams

- Fetal Movement Counts

- Amniotic fluid measurement

- Contraction Stress Tests

- Non-Stress Tests

- Biophysical Profile

Ultrasound exams:

Ultrasounds give a picture of your baby through the use of high-frequency sound waves that bounce off solid structures to create a black and white image. Ultrasounds are most commonly used to determine the baby's due date, check for twins, measure amniotic fluid volume, determine the baby's size, check the condition of the placenta and screen for some major congenital abnormalities. Not all obstetrical care providers in the U.S. offer routine ultrasounds to their clients. We, at the Department of Defense, believe that ultrasounds provide more accurate due date information and thus may be able to decrease the incidence of labor inductions and increase the detection of serious fetal problems, multiple gestations, and women at risk for placenta problems. Sometimes, when doing an ultrasound exam, the sex of your baby is obvious; but this is not always the case. Don't paint the baby's room blue or pink based on ultrasound results alone. If you don't wish to know your baby's sex, let your ultrasonographer know before the exam starts. The decision to undergo an ultrasound evaluation is entirely up to you. Ultrasounds have been used safely in obstetrics for over 25 years but there is always the remote possibility that some risk may be found in the future. If you do decide to have an ultrasound, you may want your partner to join you for your baby's first picture!

Fetal Movement Counts:

Fetal Movement Counts are a quick, easy, and inexpensive way for you to know your baby is doing well. Studies show that by recording baby's movement on a daily basis and reporting decreased movement, fetal death rates can be significantly reduced. Most authorities recommend starting fetal movement counting at 28 weeks of pregnancy. Remember to call your health care provider or Labor and Delivery if your baby has had less than ten movements in two consecutive hours or any noticeable decrease. This counting is especially important as your pregnancy progresses.

Non-Stress Tests:

Non-Stress Tests look at your baby's heart rate in response to its movement. Just as your heart rate increases with exercise, so should your baby's if all is going well. An external fetal monitor will be placed across your uterus to measure your baby's heart rate and movements. This is the same type of monitor used in the labor and delivery room. If your baby's heart rate or movement is not adequate, further testing, such as a contraction stress test or ultrasound will be done.

Contraction Stress Test:

The Contraction Stress Test uses the same fetal monitor that a Non-Stress test uses except that now you will be given some contractions and your baby's response to these contractions will be observed. If the baby reacts poorly to these very mild contractions, he or she may not tolerate real labor well. If the baby tolerates these contractions without difficulty, then we are reassured that the baby will tolerate labor.

Biophysical Profiling:

Biophysical Profiling looks at your baby's heart rate, breathing, body movements, muscle tone and amount of amniotic fluid through the use of an ultrasound. Each aspect of the test is scored and these scores are added together. The total score helps determine if it is safe for your baby to remain in your uterus.

Amniotic Fluid Measurement:

Amniotic fluid is measured through use of a limited (focusing in on just one thing) ultrasound. Adequate fluid levels tell us that your placenta is functioning adequately and that the baby is doing fine in your uterus.

True versus False Labor

Listed below are some of the differences between true and false labor. If you are not sure what you are feeling try timing your contractions with walking and with rest. If the contractions increase in intensity with walking and don't go away with rest, you are probably having true labor contractions.

True vs. False Labor

Activity	True Labor	False Labor (Braxton-Hicks)
Walking	Increases the strength of the contraction. Decreases the rest time between contractions.	Decreases strength of contraction. Increases rest time between contractions.
Strength	Contractions become more painful with time.	Contraction pain doesn't increase.
Timing: frequency & duration	Occur at regular time periods. The time from beginning to end of the contraction increases with time.	Contractions occur irregularly and the duration does not increase over time.
Location of pain	Begins in lower back and spreads to the lower abdomen and sometimes to the legs.	Stays in lower abdomen.
Cervix	Dilates (opens) & effaces (thins out, shortens).	The cervix will change positions to be in line with the vagina (from its previous posterior position) and start a small amount of dilatation and effacement to get you ready for the real thing.
Other signs	Bloody show or mucous tinged with blood occurs as cervix dilates and effaces.	No bloody show unless vaginal exam was recently performed.
Waters	Rupture (break) or leak only occurs in 15% of labors.	Don't break or leak.

Table continued on next page.

True vs. False Labor (cont.)

Activity	True Labor	False Labor *(Braxton-Hicks)*
Drinking fluids	Won't affect the frequency or duration of your contractions.	Will slow down your false contractions.
Rest	Contractions continue.	Contractions lessen or stop.

Labor & Delivery Basics

What exactly is labor and what does it do?

Labor is the term given to the entire process of bringing your baby into the world. It is certainly well named, for it is without a doubt the hardest work you will ever do. By understanding the process, knowing how to respond in a positive manner, and having a good support person, you will be ready to face your labor with confidence and knowledge.

The uterus is a muscular organ marvelously designed to house the growing fetus, and, at the appropriate time, to send him or her forth into your arms. During labor, the uterus works as a muscle by contracting and relaxing. Each uterine contraction first softens and shortens your cervix, which is the lower part of your uterus, and then opens it to allow birth to occur.

The softening and shortening of your cervix, called effacement, usually begins early in labor or even during the latter part of your pregnancy. The opening of your cervix, or dilatation commonly starts when the cervix is already soft and partially shortened or thinned out (effaced). This is especially true if this is your first baby. Women who have had prior babies may dilate a bit first, then efface and continue dilatation until delivery.

Contractions are measured from the beginning of one, to the beginning of the next, to determine the frequency and from start to finish of one contraction to measure length (duration). If you have contractions at 12:00, 12:07, 12:15 and 12:21, then your contractions are 6 to 8 minutes apart. If your contraction begins at 12:00 and ends at 12:01 then your contraction is 1 minute long. They will start out as irregular, short-lasting contractions and progress to regular, intense tightening lasting from 1 to 1½ minutes.

The hardest part of the contraction is at its peak and lasts less than 15 seconds. Remember, no matter how hard or painful they feel, they will end, usually in less than 90 seconds. Remember also, that each contraction you have puts you that much closer to holding your baby. There are many ways to cope with the pain of labor contractions and all will be explained in the labor pain section of this book.

Before labor begins:

Anytime after your 20th week of pregnancy, you may feel an irregular tightening of your uterus or Braxton-Hicks contractions. As you get closer to actual labor, this 'tightening' will become harder, more regular, and last longer. As this happens you may experience several other sensations. These include:

- **Lightening:** Your baby has dropped down into your pelvis. First time mothers experience this more. Lightening can occur 2 to 3 weeks before actual labor begins. You will notice that breathing is a lot easier but you will need to urinate even more frequently. You also may feel an increase in leg cramps, and, aching in your thighs, pelvis and lower back.

- **Engagement:** Your baby's head has passed through the upper pelvis into the lower true pelvis. This feels similar to lightening and is a sign baby is preparing for delivery. Pressure from the baby's head on the cervix will help prepare it for labor.

Preparing for Labor:

Preparation for labor should begin early in pregnancy and needs to include both physical and emotional preparation. Classes, reading, and practice will help greatly when actual labor begins.

Physical preparation: Includes staying physically fit and continuing to exercise throughout your pregnancy unless told to stop by your health care provider. Pregnancy specific exercises on a daily basis are also beneficial.

Relaxation exercises: Must be practiced with your labor coach so you both will be ready when your true contractions begin. Your coach calls the commands and checks your muscles for tension or tightness. This exercise is designed to help you remain relaxed in labor when your uterus is hard at work.

- Begin by lying on a firm surface with one or two pillows under your head and shoulders and one pillow under your knees.

- Raise arms about 2 feet from the floor or bed, stretch them slightly and hold for a few seconds, then slowly bring them down. When they are about 6 inches from the floor release your arms and let them fall limply to the floor. Legs should be fully relaxed.

- Repeat with left arm and right leg, keeping the other arm and leg totally relaxed

- Repeat with right arm and left leg, keeping the other arm and leg totally relaxed.

- Repeat with right arm and leg, keeping the other arm and leg totally relaxed.

- Repeat with left arm and leg keeping the other arm and leg totally relaxed.

- Repeat with three limbs and keep the remaining one fully relaxed.

- Learn to respond on commands such as "tighten" or "relax."

- Coach checks for tightness and relaxation.

Breathing exercises:

There is no absolute correct way to breath throughout your labor. Focused breathing is a tool to help you concentrate on your breathing and away from the pain of labor. It helps you stay relaxed and maintain control. There are many different breathing patterns to choose from. The exact breathing pattern that you use is less important than your ability to use it when the time comes. Your ability to use it will depend on how much you practiced! Listed below are some basic focused breathing techniques that you can use to help you through your labor and delivery experience. It is never too early to practice these techniques.

For early labor (1st Phase):

Take a deep cleansing breath at the start of the contraction, then breathe slowly in through your nose and out through your mouth. End the contraction with another deep cleansing breath.

Continue to breathe in this way until you feel like you need more concentrated breathing. At the point where you feel this early breathing is not helping enough, you should switch to active breathing techniques and be thinking about coming to the hospital.

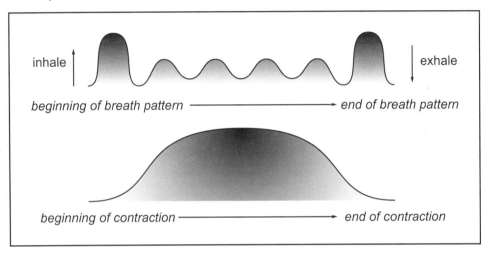

For active labor (2nd phase):

Take a deep cleansing breath at the start of the contraction, relax and stare at your focal point. Then breathe in through your mouth. "Hee" is the sound you will make as you breathe in. Follow this breath with two breaths out making the "Ha-Ha" sound. Continue the "Hee Ha-Ha" pattern until the contraction ends. At the end of the contraction take another deep cleansing breath and relax– you finished another one!

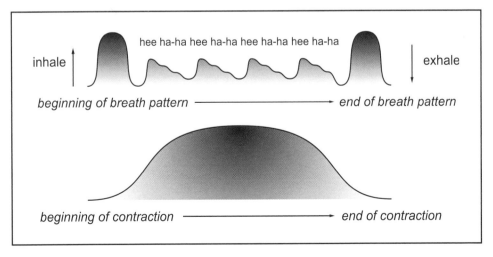

Transition breathing:

If you feel like you have to push down but are instructed not to do so, you will need to pant like a puppy or breathe quickly in and out through your mouth. This should only be to stop you from pushing (at the peak of your contraction) and for only a short period of time. If you begin to feel dizzy let your nurse know.

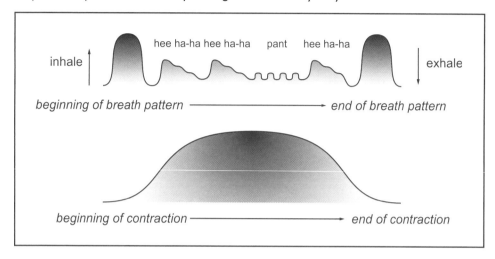

Breathing for coached pushing:

Once you are dilated and ready to push, you can either push like a bowel movement as your body tells you to or do coached pushing. The choice is usually up to you.

Coached pushing consists of starting each contraction with two-three deep cleansing breaths and holding the last one in. At the same time of your last breath, put your chin on your chest, grab your knees up and out and begin to push down (just like you are having a bowel movement). Your coach then counts slowly to ten– that is the time you will be pushing. At the count of ten, you let your breath out, take another quick and deep breath in, hold it and begin to push again. Repeat this type of breathing pattern with pushing for two to three times with each contraction. End the contraction with another deep cleansing breath and relax until the next contraction.

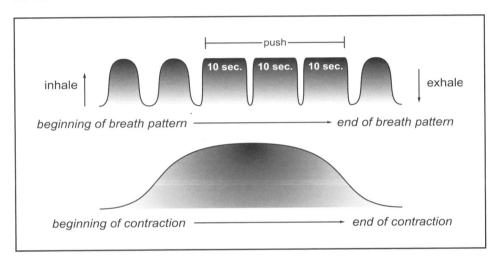

Packing for the hospital:

Around your 36th week of pregnancy you need to begin getting things packed that you wish to bring to the hospital with you. Your hospital will have gowns, slippers and robes for you to wear but if you would like to have your own make sure to pack them. It's a good idea to pack one bag for you and one for your baby. Baby's bag won't be needed for several hours or maybe not until the day after delivery. Don't bring anything too fancy or valuable.

Mom's bag:

	2 or more well fitting bras. Nursing bras may make it easier to breast-feed baby.
	2-3 pairs of cotton underwear: Bring your oldest pairs, as you will bleed quite a lot and the panties will probably get stained.
	2 or more comfortable nightgowns: If you plan to breast-feed, it will be easier if your gowns open in the front. Again, don't bring anything you don't want to get dirty.
	Slippers or slip-on shoes with non-slick soles.
	Personal care items (soap, shampoo, toothpaste, toothbrush, deodorant, comb, brush, etc.).
	Loose fitting/maternity clothing to wear home: You usually wear your maternity clothes for several days to weeks after your delivery.
	Camera with plenty of film; don't forget to check the battery!

Baby's bag:

	One going-home/picture outfit
	Car seat
	Baby bag with diapers, burp cloth, wipes for the trip home
	Blanket, hat and warm outfit if cold out

Labor tools:

	Lotion or talcum powder - for your coach to give you massages.
	Snack bag: lollipops, hard candy to suck on in labor, snack foods for coach (since you don't know when the food will be needed), and a treat for the both of you afterwards
	Lip balm or lipstick to prevent dry lips
	Something for you to concentrate on (focal point) such as a favorite picture, stuffed animal, flower, etc.
	Deck of cards to pass the time; books for you and coach
	Favorite pillow or pillows with distinctive pillow cases to identify them as yours
	Music: portable tape or CD player with a good variety of music selections
	Tennis balls in a sock for back rubs

What to do when you have false or early labor pains:

1. Keep busy and distract yourself. You can go to a movie, shopping, or find another activity that keeps your mind off these contractions.

2. Walking may help you get your labor going but if it doesn't, do NOT continue to walk until you are exhausted. Save your energy as you will need it soon.

3. Rest is important. If you are over-tired, your uterine muscles will be over-tired as well and your contractions will not be as effective as they would be if well rested. You will have the pain, but not the cervical changes!

    Try to relax by:

    a. Sipping a cup of warm milk

    b. Taking a warm (not hot) tub bath or shower

    c. Having your coach give you a back rub or body massage.

    d. Listening to some soothing music

4. Make sure you continue to drink fluids. If you become dehydrated (low in fluids), your contractions will not be as effective. You will have the pain, but not the cervical changes.

5. Don't starve yourself! Eat small amounts of easily digestible foods frequently. You have no way of knowing when your real labor will begin.

6. Stay calm. When you tense up, everything you feel will be twice as uncomfortable and labor will not progress as quickly as it should.

When to come to Labor and Delivery:

-   Rupture of Membranes- Small trickle or big gush. Note color, consistency, and time of membrane rupture. We will want to test the fluid on arrival.

-   Bright red vaginal bleeding, more than just a very small amount. Bloody show, losing your mucous plug or spotting, especially if you have had your membranes stripped recently is normal.

-   Decreased fetal movement- less than 10 movements in 2 hours after lying down and concentrating on counting

-   Severe headache

-   Difficulty seeing, blurring of vision, sparkles, or flashing lights

-   Severe swelling of your hands and face along with a sudden weight gain

-   Vomiting that continues for 24 hours

- If you are a first time mom, you will want your contractions to occur every 5 minutes for at least an hour and get stronger with walking. If you have had prior babies, you should come when your contractions are regular. You may need to come in earlier based on your individual situation which should be discussed with your health care provider.

- If unsure, come in and be checked! It's better to know than exhaust yourself with worry or come in too late.

How to tell if you are in real labor:

The first thing to remember is that every woman's labor is different. Sometimes the only way to tell if you are in labor is to go to the hospital for an exam and observation. Never feel embarrassed to call or go into the clinic or to Labor and Delivery. We are here to help you through all aspects of your pregnancy, labor, deliver and postpartum care. Please use our expertise!

What to expect when coming to Labor and Delivery:

While each medical treatment facility has a slightly different way of doing things, you can usually expect to:

1. Have a vaginal exam (if membranes are intact) to check for dilatation (opening), effacement (thinning), and station (location of baby's head).

2. Be examined for questionable rupture of membranes with a sterile speculum to avoid contamination. A small amount of fluid will be collected and put on a microscope slide to determine if it is amniotic fluid (from your bag of waters) or normal vaginal secretions. Amniotic fluid will dry on the slide in about 5 minutes forming a very distinctive fern-like pattern.

3. Have your and your baby's heartbeat timed.

4. Have your temperature, blood pressure and pulse taken.

5. Decide whether you need to be admitted now. You are usually admitted if:

    a. Your bag of waters is broken or leaking.

    b. You are 4 cm dilated.

    c. Have any potential or current problems that need close observation such as high blood pressure, fever, infection, low or high fetal heart rate, or decreased fetal movements, etc.

6. When admitted, your coach will usually need to go to the Admissions Office to complete paperwork while you will be put into a labor room.

7. Once in the labor bed you will:

    a. Be asked many personal questions.

    b. Have the external fetal monitor applied to your abdomen to measure baby's heart rate and your contractions.

c. Possibly have an IV or heparin lock inserted into a vein in your arm for a fluid access line.

d. Have lab work taken (blood and possibly urine).

8. You can ask for an enema if you are feeling uncomfortable about having a bowel movement during delivery. Many women like to avoid this and will request an enema. A small fleets enema is usually used if baby's head is engaged and/or your bag of waters is not broken.

9. Now you and your coach need to work together to have a safe and meaningful labor and birth experience.

Labor phases and how to cope:

To deliver your baby you must pass through several phases of labor. These phases include: Pre-Labor (often called false labor), early labor, active labor, and transition. At the end of these phases you will be completely dilated (10 cm) and effaced (100%) and will be ready to push your baby out into the world.

The following is a guide to each of the phases of labor, what you may feel, what you can do to help yourself, what your labor coach can do and some simple breathing techniques to help you cope with the process. The more practice time you devote to preparing yourself, the better off you, your coach and baby will be. You may want to bring your notebook with you to Labor and Delivery as a reference during labor.

Pre-Labor

Characteristics	What You May Feel	Helping Yourself	Coach's Help
Duration: hours to several days; May start and stop; Change of activity effects contractions. Not everyone feels this phase.	Abdominal or pelvic pressure, crampiness, low backache.	Relax with contractions.	Be sure to sleep and eat well.
	Burst of energy or its opposite– laziness.	Breathe normally or try slow early labor breathing.	Help with meals and chores, last minute preparations for baby.
Birthing Progress: Effacement, slight dilatation, cervical positioning.	Nesting instinct.	Don't overdo. This energy is for labor. Finish packing for hospital.	Stay in close touch. Be available for transportation.
		Eat small amounts of easily digested foods.	Encourage daily practice of breathing and relaxation techniques.
Contractions: Increased Braxton-Hicks, some uncomfortable, may begin a pattern, then fade.		Don't forget to drink fluids.	
		Pelvic rock for backache, side lying position for resting.	Help with meals and chores, last minute preparations for baby.
			Provide: – Moral support. – Entertainment. – Back massage. – Loving words.

The real thing may begin with any of the traditional labor signs. It may begin slowly (the onset of labor may not be clear to you); or may surprise you, by beginning with contractions that are strong and as close as those described under active labor. With the guidance of your health care provider, you will decide at some point in early or active labor to make the trip to the hospital.

Once there, progress will be measured by:

Effacement: thinning and softening of the cervix, measured as a percentage.

Dilation: opening of the cervix, measured in centimeters (1 to 10).

Station: the dropping down of the baby (-5 to +5 station), in relation to the pelvis

Also of interest will be what part of the baby is "presenting" (coming first through the birth canal), condition of membranes, your blood pressure, fetal heart tones, pattern of contractions, and how you are feeling!

The **First Stage,** the longest part of labor has three phases which progress from the first "real" labor contraction until the cervix is fully dilated and you start your pushing.

First Stage Labor– *Phase 1: Early Labor*

Characteristics	What You May Feel	Helping Yourself	Coach's Help
Duration: ranges from 2 hours to days.	Bubbly, excited. A little stage fright.	Enjoy this! You know your cues. Normal, light activity, plenty of rest.	This phase is usually spent at home and you will need to be in close contact in case she needs you.
Birthing Progress: Cervix dilates to 4 cm.	Wish to tell the world.		
	Gradually less sociable, more serious, beginning to realize it's work.	Relax and breathe thru contraction; use good positioning.	Stay in touch hourly.
Contractions: Last 30-60 seconds; are 5-15 minutes apart, and are mild but definite; progressively longer, stronger, closer together.		Call the L&D unit.	Support, entertainment.
	Wavelike pressure/ crampiness in back or front- all over tummy or very low in the tummy with contractions.	Pelvic rock for backache, slow breathing for each contraction. Warm shower.	Extra rest for you too.
			Call sitter for older children.
		Clear liquids, if allowed. Light, small snacks.	Encourage relaxation.
	Hungry, thirsty, "time to get going."		Start coaching breathing exercises just for practice.
			Hand on tummy to get acquainted with contractions.
			Back massage if needed.
			When she needs to concentrate on breathing, begin to time each contraction.
			Watch for change of attitude.
			Offer fluids often.
			Carefully drive to hospital when she is ready.

For early labor
(1st Phase Breathing):

inhale — exhal
beginning of breath pattern ———— end of breath patter

beginning of contraction ———— end of contraction

First Stage Labor– *Phase 2: Active Labor*

Characteristics	What You May Feel	Helping Yourself	Coach's Help
Duration: 4-8 hours. **Birthing Progress:** Cervix dilates from 4 to 8 cm. **Contractions:** Last 45-75 seconds and are 3-5 minutes apart and are quite strong, peak more quickly.	Serious, need to concentrate. Intense pressure with contractions. Vaginal bleeding Backache may intensify or vanish. Trembling legs. Flushed warm, dry mouth. Nausea Discouraged if no progress. Very self-centered.	Focal point away from traffic pattern in room. Switch to focused breathing. Urinate often. Change position. May want to suck on lollipop. Tell others of needs! Turn on background music. Walk or shower if possible. Try squatting or sitting on exercise ball.	Be prepared with information for admissions if not pre-admitted. Return quickly to labor and delivery. Time contractions. Talk her thru them. Check for relaxation and help get her to relax. Anticipate needs for comfort and handle distractions. Walk with her if able. Help her to bathroom often (tell nurses). Help her change positions often. Tell nurses if she has urge to push. Massage. Praise! Encourage often!

For active labor
(2nd Phase Breathing):

hee ha-ha hee ha-ha hee ha-ha hee ha-ha

inhale ↑   ↓ exhale

beginning of breath pattern ⟶ *end of breath pattern*

beginning of contraction ⟶ *end of contraction*

First Stage Labor– *Phase 3: Transition*

Characteristics	What You May Feel	Helping Yourself	Coach's Help
Duration: 15 minutes to 1½ hours. **Birthing Progress:** Cervix dilates from 7-8 to 10 cm. **Contractions:** 60-90 seconds long, 2-3 minutes apart. Very strong, tremendous pressure, may have more than one peak.	Confused, irritable, not wanting to be touched, afraid of losing control. Increased rectal pressure. Urge to bear down, very tired and sleepy. Nausea, vomiting, burps, shaky legs, or trembling all over, leg cramps. Hiccups, dizziness, tingling hands and face (hyperventilation). More vaginal discharge caused by descent of baby. Hot and perspiring, or cold and shivering. Increased backache as baby descends.	Switch to transition breathing pattern; take each contraction one at a time. DON'T push! Pant or blow till urge has passed. Concentrate on relaxing, especially between contractions. Try to keep breathing slow - don't hyperventilate. Ask to change bed pads if needed. Change positions often. Urinate often. Stay in bed. Rest between contractions-many women fall asleep between them.	Be firm in coaching, never mind her mood. She'll thank you later for coaching breathing. Put your face about 10 inches in front of her face and do the breathing exercise if she is having difficulty in maintaining control and breathing. If she doesn't want to be touched, back off—this is only temporary—but keep on coaching her breathing though the contractions. Coach her to pant or blow if she starts to push and call your nurse. Let her sleep between contractions-keep distractions down, dim the lights, lower the sound. Wake her at onset of each contraction (watch monitor) and start her breathing. Have cool cloth for face, lips and mouth ready.

First Stage Labor– *Phase 3: Transition (cont.)*

Characteristics	What You May Feel	Helping Yourself	Coach's Help
			Stroke legs, back, and shoulders if it helps her relax.
			Straighten limb and flex foot to relieve leg cramps.
			Remind her she is getting closer to holding her baby!
			Help her get into different positions often.
			Make sure she is urinating often.
			Ask staff about getting ready for delivery.
			PRAISE!

Transition breathing:

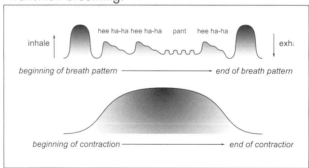

The **Second Stage** includes the time from full dilation of the cervix until the baby is born. Setup for delivery will begin now if it is not your first baby.

Second Stage Labor– *Pushing*

Characteristics	What You May Feel	Helping Yourself	Coach's Help
Duration: Varies greatly- 2 pushes to 2 hours.	Urge to push varies, usually strong.	Take two cleansing breaths, and rest between contractions.	Check her position and help her to change it frequently.
Birthing Progress: Pushing the baby down the birth canal and out into the world.	Great relief to push.	Listen closely to coaching from team.	Remind her of cleansing breaths at beginning and end of each contraction.
	May feel uncertain at first but you will soon get into it.		Encourage long pushes.
			Let her rest/ sleep between contractions.
			Keep distractions to a minimum.
			Wet her forehead, lips and mouth with cool wet cloth.
			Give ice chips between pushes.
			Ask for mirror to increase motivation.
			Respect her mood. She may be quiet, bubbly or crabby. Remember she is working really hard.
Coached breathing:			Coach firmly.

push

10 sec. 10 sec. 10 sec.

inhale   exha

beginning of breath pattern ———————→ end of breath pattern

beginning of contraction ———————→ end of contraction

Second Stage Labor– *Pushing (cont.)*

Characteristics	What You May Feel	Helping Yourself	Coach's Help
Contraction: Last 60-90 seconds and are 2-5 minutes apart, peak more slowly than transition contractions, and may have more rest breaks between.	Alertness returns, new burst of energy.	Enjoy the excitement.	Support her during pushes.
	Back pain may vanish or return.	Pushing harder may help you to cope with pain.	Limit movement. Stay next to or behind her head now unless told otherwise.
	Great pressure in rectum. Stretching, stinging sensation around vagina as crowning approaches; numb for birth of baby.	Release perineum as completely as you can and think "Open, baby out!"	Remind her to "Relax her bottom."
		Lie back and pant or blow for birth of baby's head.	Support her head and shoulders so she may watch baby emerge.
	Actual feel of baby emerging is warm and pleasant relief!	Push as directed for baby's shoulders.	Look to see WHO'S HERE!
		Get ready to hold your new baby.	If this has been discussed and planned: Get ready to cut cord.
			Get the camera out and ready for first shot of new baby.
			Welcome your baby into the world!

The **Third Stage** includes the time from baby's birth to expulsion of the afterbirth.

Third Stage Labor

What is Happening	What You May Feel	Helping Yourself	Coach
Duration: up to 30 minutes. **Birthing Progress:** Afterbirth comes out (placenta, membrane, cord). **Contractions:** Few, mild ones.	May or may not notice contractions. Chilled, shivery, impatient. Overwhelmed and overjoyed!	Ask to push placenta out yourself. Respond to coaching. Nursing baby stimulates your uterus to contract. Concentrate on your baby.	Reinforce instructions. Remind her to relax. Enjoy watching or holding your baby. Stay near until she is ready to rest.

Pain management in labor:

Each woman will respond differently to her contractions. This response depends on many factors to include:

- Time spent in labor
- Level of pain tolerance
- Quality of coaching
- Emotional and physical state
- Preparation for labor
- Size and position of baby
- Stage of labor

Coping techniques:

Since it is impossible to predict how your labor will go and how well you will cope with your labor, it is very important for you to know all your options. The absolute safest option for you and your baby is to not rely on any medications while in labor. Unfortunately, this is not always possible. If you require medications after trying the various non-medication techniques listed below, your health care provider will determine the safest route, amount, and timing of the medication.

- **Breathing with the contractions:** Various breathing techniques are taught in childbirth preparation classes and it doesn't matter which one you choose to use. By using these breathing techniques you will be focusing on breathing and not on the pain of your contractions. Simple but effective breathing techniques are outlined in the Phases of Labor section.

- **Medications:** There are several different medications that can be given in labor to help cope with the contraction pain. How much, when to give the medication and what to give depends on many factors. Your health care provider will work with you to minimize the pain as much as is safe for you and your baby. There is no labor medication that is guaranteed to be 100% free of side effects, although with proper monitoring, dosing and timing of medications, side effects can be kept to a minimum.

  - **Analgesics:** Narcotics and synthetic narcotics- these can be given through a shot in your muscle or into your IV to dull the pain and help you to relax. IV medications act quickly but don't last as long as an injection into a muscle. We try not to give these medications within an hour of delivery to prevent the baby from being born with the drug. If baby comes quicker than expected then a narcotic blocking medication can be given to your baby to block its effects. Other side effects include slowing of your labor or stopping it if given too soon.

  - **Spinal Block:** A narcotic or local anesthetic is injected into the spine to numb you from your waist downward. These are commonly used for cesarean sections. Side effects include: itching, failure to block the pain, severe headaches, or slowed breathing.

  - **Epidural:** A small plastic tube containing a diluted narcotic and local anesthetic is inserted in your spine. The medicine in the tubing bathes the spines which causes numbness in your lower half of your body. It takes about 10 to 20 minutes to work and can be adjusted as your labor progresses. Possible side effects include decrease in your uterine contractions, prolonged labor, lower blood pressure and decrease in the baby's circulation, urine retention, no relief in your pain, spinal nerve damage (rarely permanent), low back pain after delivery, and increased chance of cesarean section especially if given early in labor. The tubing occasionally falls out of place and needs to be replaced. The anesthetic medicine can enter your blood stream and you may become light headed, confused or have convulsions. This almost never happens. Rarely, the medicine can also enter the spinal fluid, which could lead to a higher degree of numbness or muscle weakness requiring help with breathing and/or blood pressure. Epidurals will take away up to 80% of your pain but will not take away your feelings of pressure from the baby. It can also be used if forceps, vacuum assistance or cesarean delivery is needed.

Why a Cesarean Section (C/S)?

There are several reasons to perform a cesarean section and often times it is a combination of reasons that help make the final decision. It is never performed strictly to avoid labor contractions as this is a major surgical procedure. Unless it is an emergency situation in which a delay could harm either you or your baby, the doctor performing the surgery will explain to you why a cesarean is needed.

Reasons for cesarean births include:

- **Cephalic-pelvic disproportion (CPD):** Baby is too big or your pelvis is too small to allow for your baby to be born through your birth canal.

- **Fetal distress:** Baby's heartbeat is slowing down to a dangerous level and won't come back to normal levels despite usual interventions such as increased fluids, oxygen and position change.

- **Excessive vaginal bleeding**

- **Active Herpes or diseases that could affect your baby**

- **Malposition or malpresentation:** Baby is in an unsafe position such as breech, or unsafe presentation such as neck fully extended that will not allow him/ her to be born safely through the birth canal.

- **Failure to progress:** The cervix is not dilating (opening) properly even with adequate period of time with strong contractions.

- **Placenta previa:** Placenta is covering all or part of the cervical opening leading to severe vaginal bleeding.

- **Placenta abruption:** Placenta separates from the uterine wall and blocks oxygen exchange to your baby.

- **Previous cesarean section:** especially if you had a previous classical incision (runs up and down your abdomen). Often even if you had a cesarean previously, you can still attempt to deliver vaginally this time.

What usually happens with a C/S?

- You will be counseled as to why a C/S is needed and you will sign a consent form allowing the C/S to occur.

- You will have an IV (tube into vein) and Foley catheter (tube in bladder) inserted.

- You will be counseled on what type of anesthetic is best for you and baby.

  - General anesthesia (you go to sleep)

  - Regional anesthesia (you are numb from waist down)

- The operating room can be quite crowded with nurses, doctors and assistants. Depending on the situation, your partner may be allowed to accompany you. Ask your doctor. In the operating room, you will be placed on the operating table. Once on the table, your abdomen and pubic area will be washed, shaved and drapes or covers will be placed over your abdomen. The anesthetist will administer the anesthesia after taking several blood pressure readings and monitoring your other vital signs (respiration rate, temperature). After the anesthesia begins to work, a cut will be made below your belly button to get the baby out. You will not be able to see this incision, even if awake, because a drape will be between your head and your abdomen to block your view. After the baby is born, the pediatrician will make sure baby is OK and then let you hold/ see baby depending on your baby's condition. After your abdomen is sutured, you will be taken to a recovery area for several hours. You will be very sleepy at this time. When you are fully recovered you will be taken to the Postpartum area to begin your life with your new baby.

After a C/S can I deliver vaginally?

In many cases you can deliver vaginally after having a C/S. Your doctor or midwife will help you decide if a vaginal birth is safe for you.

Many of our patients have specific requests for management during labor and delivery. Our goal for managing your labor and delivery is to help you bring your baby into this world in a safe and friendly environment. We hope this will be a wonderful experience for you.

Most published "birth plans" provide a menu of options with check boxes for things that you want during labor and delivery. These forms suggest that having a baby is like having a meal at a smorgasbord, pick what you want for each course the price is the same. However, when it comes to labor, some of these "menu items" are more expensive (have more risk) than others. Below we provide you some information about our common practices and reasons for them. If you have any special requests or would like to discuss any of these issues further, please make a note of them below and we will discuss them with you.

Environment—if you would like to have the lights down, or bring/play your own music, that is usually acceptable and is simply a matter of conveying your desire to the staff caring for you while on Labor and Delivery. During the actual delivery or after the delivery if stitching is required, some lighting is necessary.

Visitors—Your partner is welcome throughout your labor and delivery unless an emergency cesarean section is necessary and you have to have general anesthesia. In addition, depending upon your wishes, their maturity, the room size and your condition, other family members/friends are usually allowed to attend the birthday party.

Pain management—Except in specific circumstances, we usually leave the type of pain management up to you. Available options include, Lamaze-type techniques (no medications), IV narcotics and regional anesthetics (such as an epidural). All options for pain relief have their own risks and benefits. We base the type and timing of pain relief methods on your wishes and individual situation.

IV—We strongly recommend that you have an IV in place during labor so that you can more quickly be cared for in the event of an emergency. It is common to attach the IV to tubing and give some IV fluids but this can usually be limited if you desire.

Food and Drink—We recommend limiting intake to clear liquids and hard candy so that your stomach can be relatively empty. If an emergency delivery is necessary and you have to have general anesthesia, it is much safer for you if your stomach is empty.

Monitors—We usually do continuous fetal monitoring once you are admitted to labor and delivery. If your pregnancy is uncomplicated and the initial fetal monitoring is reassuring and there is adequate nursing staff available, it may be appropriate to go for periods of time without fetal monitors in place. Usually the fetal monitors are placed on your abdomen over your uterus. If additional information is necessary we sometime put monitors directly on the baby or inside your uterus.

Labor positions—As long as we can monitor the baby often enough to be sure that the baby is OK (varies with the situation), you can move around the room if you would like.

Delivery positions—Most women deliver while lying on their back or side and most providers have the most experience delivering babies from this position. If you would like to deliver in an alternative fashion, please let us know.

Episiotomy—We do not routinely cut episiotomies. If they are performed it is usually because we need to get the baby out quickly.

Forceps and Vacuums—We do not use forceps or vacuums without a reason. Vacuum or forceps assisted delivery is recommended when your cervix is completely dilated but the baby needs to be delivered more quickly than you are able to push the baby out or because you have been unable to make enough progress on your own. If forceps or vacuum is recommended it is because the provider believes that the potential benefits of the procedure outweigh the risks.

The umbilical cord—If you desire, your partner can cut the cord unless, the baby needs extra help transitioning to life outside of the womb and we have to move quickly.

Bonding—You can let us know at the time if you prefer to have the baby placed on your abdomen right after birth or have the baby cleaned off first and then given to you. Unless there is a medical reason to do otherwise, we keep the mom and baby together after the delivery.

Feeding—Usually the best time to begin breast-feeding is shortly after birth. We support and encourage this practice.

Medications for baby—We typically give the baby a shot of vitamin K in the thigh and put some antibiotic ointment on the eyes within the first half an hour after birth. These medications help the baby's blood to clot properly and decrease the risk of eye infections that the baby may acquire during the birth. If you would rather the medications be given later or not at all, please let us know.

Please share with us any of your concerns or special requests.

_____

_____

_____

_____

_____

_____

Remember in the event of an emergency regarding your health or the health of your unborn baby, we will do our best to keep you informed but we may need to modify your birth plan.

Baby Equipment for the First Week

The following is a list of baby items that will be very helpful to have prior to bringing baby home. Give the list to friends when they ask what you need or at least leave it around in convenient areas for them to see.

Infant car seat:

- You will need a rear facing car seat to bring your baby home from the hospital. Make sure you know how to install it safely into your car's backseat. Your baby won't be discharged without one.

Clothing:

- 4-6 shirts, sleepers and gowns. Plan on at least a few change of clothes a day due to spit up and other mishaps.
- Warm clothes such as hats, blankets, booties, etc. if needed.

Bedding:

- Some type of crib or bassinet: Make sure the slats are no farther apart than 2 inches (6 cm).
- 4-5 blankets and sheets.

Bathing/diaper supplies:

- 2-3 towels, 4 wash cloths.
- 3-4 dozen diapers (disposable or cloth). Plan on your baby using about a dozen/day.
- Baby shampoo and soap.
- Saline nose drops.
- Baby bath or pad for sink.
- Baby hairbrush or comb.
- Baby fingernail clippers or scissors.
- Mild laundry soap.
- Cotton swabs or cotton balls.
- Soft cloths or disposable wipes for cleaning after diaper change.
- Petroleum jelly or other lubricating jelly.

Baby first aid:

- Digital or rectal thermometer, baby Acetaminophen and rubbing alcohol.

Breast-feeding supplies:

- 5-6 handkerchiefs, clean cloths, or breast pads for leaking breasts.
- 2-3 nursing bras.
- Nursing tops and nightgowns for added convenience.

Bottle-feeding supplies:

- 8 (4 ounce) baby bottles, caps and nipples.
- Bottle and nipple brush for cleaning.
- 1 quart measuring cup.

Extras you might want:

- Baby bag to carry all this in.
- Pacifiers.
- Few cloth diapers for burping cloths and clean-ups.
- Wet wipes to carry in diaper bag.
- Changing mat.

Sex after delivery:

It is best to avoid sex for at least 3-6 weeks following the delivery of your baby in order to give yourself time to recover from the changes associated with childbirth. Your stitches (if you had any) should be totally dissolved and your vaginal discharge greatly reduced by this time showing that you are well on your way to complete recovery. The perineal area (or area between the vagina and the rectum) will still be slightly tender but that doesn't mean that healing isn't taking place. In order to help make your first sexual experience after the delivery an enjoyable one, there are a few helpful hints that we suggest you follow:

- Have your partner or yourself apply gentle pressure at the entrance of your vagina towards your rectum. If this is very painful, it is better to wait until it does not cause discomfort before having sex.

- Use a lubricant such as K-Y Jelly® around the entrance of your vagina as you may be drier for a period of time following your delivery. This is especially true if you are breast-feeding.

- The side position may be more comfortable if you had a midline episiotomy. This position places less pressure on the suture area.

- Make sure baby is asleep so you'll be less likely to be disturbed.

- If you are breast-feeding, you may wish to keep your bra on in order to absorb the milk that can be released during your orgasm.

- Be sure to use some form of birth control. You can become pregnant at any time after delivery. You release the egg 2 weeks before your period. You usually won't know when your egg is being released.

- Be sure to spend time together as a couple even if you're not quite ready to have intercourse.

Masters and Johnson, the primary experts on sexuality, have found that women in the first 2 months after delivery were slower to respond to sexual stimulation and responded less strongly. In spite of this, women did not find sex less enjoyable. Just remember, you must be ready both physically and mentally before resuming sex. Don't rush it. There are many other ways to express your love.

Birth control methods after delivery:

Before resuming sexual intercourse, we recommend waiting until your bleeding has stopped, or at least greatly decreased, your stitches (if you had any) have healed and you are on a reliable form of birth control. Ideally it would be best to wait until your 6-8 week postpartum appointment to make sure everything is healing without problems and that your birth control method is adequate. If you feel well enough to enjoy sex prior to that time, there are many birth control options to choose from.

If you are not breast-feeding, you can expect to have your first period anywhere from 4 to 6 weeks after the delivery. With full breast-feeding (no supplements of any kind) your periods may be delayed up to six months. Unfortunately you will release your egg (and therefore are fertile) before your first period whenever it occurs. It is because of this that we recommend all women have a reliable type of birth control prior to resuming intercourse, no matter when the intercourse occurs. Luckily, there are several good choices of reliable birth control methods available for both breast-feeding and non-breast-feeding women.

Non-hormonal methods:

Condoms and foam are excellent methods for women after delivery. These methods avoid the very small possibility of hormones effecting breast-feeding. The small risk of blood clots right after delivery is avoided. Barrier methods include:

- **Withdrawal:** The man pulls his penis out of the vagina before he "comes" to keep the sperm from getting to the egg. This takes great self control, experience and trust. Effectiveness is only around 81% but increases greatly when a condom is used as well.

- **Spermicides (foam, cream, tablets, suppositories and film):** Chemicals that are applied in the vagina less than one hour before sex. Much more effective if used with a barrier method.

- **Male condoms:** Offers protection against infection. This is especially important in the post-partum period when your uterine wall is healing. To be effective, your partner needs to use these each and every time.

- **Female condoms:** Plastic tube that lines the vagina to prevent sperm from reaching the cervix. This method also protects against Sexually Transmitted Diseases (STDs). These are not intended for use with a male condom. You will need to choose one or the other.

- **Diaphragm and spermicidal jelly or cream:** A soft rubber cup that covers the cervix and thereby blocks sperm from entering the uterus. Should be used with a spermicidal jelly or cream. Must be used prior to each and every time you have sex. You must be fitted for this device (even if you have one from before this pregnancy) at your postpartum visit. A diaphragm is left in place no shorter than 6 hours after sex and no longer than 24 hours. For each additional act of intercourse you must apply new spermicide. Do NOT remove the diaphragm when adding new spermicide.

- **Cervical cap and spermicidal jelly or cream:** A soft rubber cup similar to the diaphragm but smaller. Should be used with a spermicidal jelly or cream. Must be used prior to each and every time you have sex. You must be fitted for this device (even if you have an old one) at your postpartum visit. You leave this in place no shorter than 6 hours after sex and no longer than 48 hours. You can use the cervical cap for up to 48 hours of protection.

- **Intrauterine device (IUD):** Small, flexible plastic frame inserted into the uterus through the vagina. These are effective up to 10 years depending on type. If you would like this method, discuss it with your health care provider prior to your postpartum visit so arrangements can be made for its insertion postpartum.

- **Permanent sterilization:** A woman can obtain a tubal ligation or a man can have a vasectomy; if you are absolutely sure you do not ever want future children. This method is over 99% effective. Institutions will vary on requirements needed (usually age and number of children) to have this procedure performed. If this interests you, talk to your health care provider early on in your pregnancy. Tubal ligation can often be done prior to leaving the hospital, if arranged for in advance.

Lactational Amenorrhea Method (LAM) for breast-feeding women:

This method provides some protection against pregnancy for up to 6 months postpartum if no supplements are added to the baby's diet and intervals between breast-feeding do not exceed 4 hours during the day and 6 hours at night. The use of a condom with foam and or withdrawal increases effectiveness.

Hormonal methods:

Breast-feeding options: It is recommended that breast-feeding women avoid using combined oral contraceptives (those that have both estrogen and progesterone) since they may decrease the milk supply and alter the milk composition. Studies have shown varied results but most report a decline in the mineral content of the breast milk with use of combined oral contraceptives. Even though existing evidence (scant that it is) suggests that the combined oral contraceptives do not directly harm infants, most providers feel safer using the progesterone-only birth control methods if hormonal contraception is desired. Studies have shown no ill effects of progesterone-only methods on lactation and some studies have suggested there may even be a slight increase in milk volume. Progesterone-only methods include:

- **Progesterone only pills (POPs or minipills):** It may be best to wait until 6 weeks after delivery since there is a theoretical (unproven) risk that POPs may pose a problem to your baby. This theoretical risk is based on your newborn's liver and kidneys not being fully developed and therefore unable to break down and excrete drugs. If the need is great and you are willing to take this theoretical risk, then ask your health care provider for a supply prior to leaving the hospital. You should wait until your milk supply is well established before to starting. The amount of progesterone is even lower than the amount found in low dose combination pills.

- **Progesterone injection:** This method is a liquid form of progesterone and is very effective in preventing pregnancy for 12 weeks. Several medical treatment facilities will give this injection prior to discharge from the hospital.

Hormonal options for women who are bottle-feeding: Combined oral contraceptives can be started 2 weeks after delivery. Waiting the two weeks allows for the recommended vaginal rest and avoids the period of peak risk for postpartum blood clots.

- **Progesterone injection:** A progesterone injection given prior to discharge from the hospital is effective immediately and lasts for 12 weeks from date of injection.

- **Progesterone only pills (POPs):** Prescribed for women who wish to avoid the estrogen found in combined oral contraceptives.

- **Combined hormonal injection such as Lunelle®:** an injection given every four weeks containing both estrogen and progesterone.

Methods that don't work well enough to depend on:

- Breast-feeding: if you miss any feedings, are ill, baby gone etc. you could ovulate and become pregnant.

- Feminine hygiene products

- Douching.

- Urinating after sex.

- Withdrawal of the penis.

- Fertility awareness immediately after delivery.

- When in doubt, check with your health care provider.

Effectiveness and Side Effects of Various Birth Control Methods:

Method	% Pregnant within the First Year	Advantages	Side Effects
No Birth Control Used	85 out of 100		Pregnancy and no protection against STDs.
Pill: (Oral Contraceptive Pill) Progestin only or Estrogen & Progesterone combined pills	5 out of 100 1 out of 100 1 out of 100	Easy to use and very effective. Periods are usually lighter, regular with less pain. Studies have shown women using the Pill have less ovarian and uterine cancer in later life, less acne, less Premenstrual Symptoms, less anemia (iron poor blood).	**POPs (mini pills):** Irregular bleeding, weight gain, breast tenderness, less protection against ectopic pregnancy. **Combined:** Dizziness, nausea, changes in menstruation, mood, and weight; rarely, cardiovascular disease, including high blood pressure, blood clots, heart attack, and strokes. Serious side effects very rare. Neither pill protects against STDs.
Intra-Uterine Devices	Less than 1 out of 100	Effective up to 10 years depending on type. Don't have to think about it before sex.	Pain, bleeding, infection, other post-surgical complications. No protection against STDs.
Progesterone Injections	Less than 1 out of 100	Usually no periods after a few months. May help breast-feeding women have more milk.	Irregular bleeding, weight gain, breast tenderness, headaches. No protection against STDs.

Table continued on next page.

Effectiveness and Side Effects of Various Birth Control Methods
(cont.)

Method	% Pregnant within the First Year	Advantages	Side Effects
Combined hormone injections	Less than 1 out of 100	Once a month injection. Fertile in about 2-4 months after stopping injections. Advantages similar to the birth control pill.	Changes in menstrual cycle, weight gain. Similar to oral contraceptives–combined type. Serious side effects very rare. No protection against STDs.
Male condoms	12 out of 100	Protection against most STDs. Can use as soon after delivery as needed. Inexpensive and doesn't require a prescription.	Irritation and allergic reactions (less likely with polyurethane), must use with each time, can break or fall off. Should use with spermicides.
Female condoms	21 out of 100	Protection against most STDs. Can use as soon after delivery as needed. Inexpensive and doesn't require a prescription.	Irritation and allergic reactions (less likely with polyurethane), must use with each time, can break or fall off. Should use with spermicides.
Diaphragm with spermicide	21 out of 100	No drugs or chemicals are absorbed into the body. Doesn't affect your period.	Irritation and allergic reactions, urinary tract infection. Risk of Toxic Shock Syndrome, a rare but serious infection, when kept in place longer than recommended. No protection against STDs.

Table continued on next page.

Effectiveness and Side Effects of Various Birth Control Methods (cont.)

Method	% Pregnant within the First Year	Advantages	Side Effects
Cervical cap Women with children Women without children	36 out of 100 18 out of 100	No drugs or chemicals are absorbed into the body. Doesn't affect your period.	Irritation and allergic reactions, abnormal Pap test. Risk of Toxic Shock Syndrome, a rare but serious infection when kept in place longer than recommended. No protection against STDs.
Vaginal Ring	1-2 out of 100	Place into vagina for three weeks then remove. You don't have to worry about taking pill every day, getting an injection or using something prior to sex each time.	Male may feel it with sex. Can't store in hot location; it releases hormone. No protection against STDs.
Spermicides	26 out of 100	Inexpensive and don't need a prescription. Much more effective if used with a barrier method (condom, diaphragm, cervical cap).	Irritation and allergic reactions, urinary tract infections. No protection against STDs.
Withdrawal	19 out of 100	Nothing to buy, inject or put on.	Takes lot of self-control, presence of sperm in fluid prior to ejaculation. Not effective. No protection against STDs.

Table continued on next page.

Effectiveness and Side Effects of Various Birth Control Methods
(cont.)

Method	% Pregnant within the First Year	Advantages	Side Effects
Fertility awareness (Natural Family Planning)	3 out of 100 (if done daily and accurately)	No physical health risks to its use and can also be used to get pregnant. Need to know how to record daily basal body temperature and note cervical mucous.	Difficult to learn this method after delivery because your cycles will not be regular. Involves careful checking and recording of daily body signs. No protection against STDs.
Male sterilization: Vasectomy	0.15 out of 100	Done only once and highly effective.	Pain, bleeding, infection, other minor post surgical complications. No protection against STDs.
Female sterilization: Tubal Ligation	0.5 out of a 100	Done only once and highly effective.	Pain, bleeding, infection, other post-surgical complications. No protection against STDs.
Emergency contraceptives (morning after pills)	Reduces pregnancy from single episode by 80%	Only method that can be used after intercourse to prevent a pregnancy. Effective as a back-up method to other methods.	Nausea, vomiting, abdominal pain, fatigue, headache. No protection against STDs.
Evra® patch	1 out of 100	Once a week patch. Ability to become pregnant quickly returns when stopped. Advantages similar to the birth control pill.	Similar to oral contraceptives-combined pill. Less effective for women over 198 pounds. Skin irritation. No protection against STDs.

Table continued on next page.

Effectiveness and Side Effects of Various Birth Control Methods (cont.)

Method	% Pregnant within the First Year	Advantages	Side Effects
Lactation Amenorrhea Method (LAM)	2 out of 100	Nothing to take therefore no risks to baby or you.	Only effective if not giving supplements, and feeding every 4 hours in the day and every 6 hours at night. Much more effective if used with condoms, or other barrier methods.

Listing of medications/drugs does not represent endorsement by VA/DoD

Breast-feeding

Among the many things you must consider before you deliver is how you will feed your infant(s). More and more mothers are choosing to breast-feed, because it is one of the most important contributors to a baby's health. Additional benefits are that breast-feeding helps you feel healthier and saves money. Breast-feeding is recommended for at least the first year of a baby's life, but many studies have shown that any amount of breast-feeding is beneficial. It is important to know that there are a number of resources available to help you succeed.

Learning as much as you can about breast-feeding early in your pregnancy is the best preparation. The more comfortable you feel with breast-feeding, the easier it will be for you. There are a number of books, pamphlets, and web based resources you can use. Ask your doctor or the nursing staff in the clinic for information regarding local lactation resources.

Benefits to Mom:

- Breast-feeding relaxes you – when you breast feed, hormones are released which calm and relax you.

- Breast-feeding saves money by reducing or eliminating the cost of buying formula.

- Breast-feeding reduces health care costs.

- Breast-feeding decreases the incidence and/or severity of specific illnesses in infants.[1]

- Breast-feeding is convenient – no mixing, measuring.

- Breast-feeding uses up extra calories, so it makes it easier to lose the pounds you gained during your pregnancy.

- Breast-feeding helps the uterus to get back to its original size and lessens any bleeding you may have after giving birth.

- Breast-feeding can help you bond with your baby - physical contact is important to a newborn and can help them feel more secure, warm and comforted.

Benefits to Baby:

- Breast fed babies have a healthier start in life, because breast milk contains all the nutrients baby needs, regardless of whether your baby is premature or full term.

- Breast milk has the perfect mix of nutrients for your baby's digestive system.

- Breast milk protects a baby from many illnesses such as diarrhea, ear infections, respiratory tract infections, diabetes, urinary tract infections, and severe bacterial infections.[2]

- Breast milk is always the right temperature for your baby.

- Breast fed babies are less likely to become overweight.

- Breast-feeding promotes the proper development of jaw and facial structures.

- Breast milk aids in the development of baby's brain and nervous system.

Myths and Truths:

There are many myths or "old wives tales" and breast-feeding has more than its share of them. Listed on the next page are just a few of the more common *myths* that you may have heard and the truth behind them.

Breast-feeding Myths and Truths

Myth	Truth
You need large breasts to make enough milk.	Shape and size is due to the layers of muscle and fat. Size has no effect on milk production.
You can't work and breast-feed.	Breast milk can be expressed and stored for feeding the baby while you are at work.
You can't smoke and breast-feed.	The American Academy of Pediatrics states that it is better to breast-feed than formula-feed even if you smoke. If you do smoke, try to cut down as much as possible (less than 6 cigarettes a day). Don't smoke right before breast-feeding and never smoke in the house or anywhere around the baby. Second-hand smoke increases the incidence of pneumonia, bronchitis and SIDS in your baby.
You can't use birth control and breast-feed.	There are several birth control methods that are safe for breast-feeding women, such as condoms, foam, diaphragms, and birth control pills that contain progesterone (mini-pill).
You can't become pregnant while breast-feeding.	Exclusive breast-feeding (no pacifiers or bottles) can delay ovulation for some women. The Lactational Amenorrhea Method (LAM) is more effective when used with another birth control method such as condom. If you plan to use this method of birth control, talk with your health care provider for details.
You will be tied down.	A breast-fed baby is very portable. You don't have to carry extra gear with you. If you return to work or need to be away from your baby, you can express milk for a baby sitter.
You must drink milk to make milk.	Cow's milk is an inexpensive source of calcium and protein. You can get calcium by eating dairy products, collards, canned salmon, calcium enriched tofu, and juices. Other good protein sources are meats, eggs, peanut butter, and soy/tofu.
Each member of the family has to feed the baby to bond too.	Bonding can occur in a variety of ways such as: cuddling, playing, holding, talking or reading to and rocking the baby.

Diet:

- Eat well to feel well

- You only need 200 calories more a day than your pre-pregnancy diet

- You need 1200mg Calcium a day

- You need 3 or more servings of protein a day

- Drink 8-12 glasses of non-caffeinated fluids a day

You do not have to avoid any particular food, unless you have a family history of allergy (shellfish, citrus, dairy, etc). You may eat anything you are used to eating. If your baby is fussy, it does not mean he is allergic to your milk. Babies can be sensitive to something you have eaten. Do not start eliminating foods from your diet. The most common food sensitivity is an excess intake of cow's milk. You may want to reduce or eliminate milk from your diet and see how baby reacts. Usually baby will improve within 1-3 days.

Supplies:

Several good nursing bras:

These will support your breasts and make breast-feeding a lot more convenient. It is recommended that you buy your nursing bras in the last month or two of your pregnancy when your breasts have already increased in size. When you buy your bras, make sure they're all-cotton, they fit comfortably around your rib cage when fastened on the loose setting, and there is extra room in the cup. A tight bra is uncomfortable and can cause sore nipples, plugged ducts, and breast infections. When trying on nursing bras, make sure you can open the nursing flap with one hand (so you won't have to put baby down each time you feed). Purchase one or two bras to see if you like them, then buy more as needed.

Nursing Shirts:

Most maternity stores sell clever nursing shirts. These shirts are great, because they are attractive, most people don't know that they are for nursing, and they make it easier to breast feed while you are learning. Some mothers are comfortable wearing large T-shirts. Button front tops and two-piece sets also work well once you're comfortable with breast-feeding.

Nursing Pads:

These are placed in your bra to protect your bra and clothes. At the beginning, many mothers experience periodic leaking of their breast milk. Nursing pads may only be needed the first few weeks.

Pumps:

A pump is useful to have for a few reasons. You may need to be away from your baby for short time periods, so you'll need to provide your baby sitter with some breast milk to feed your baby(ies). If you plan to return to work, you'll need to pump your breasts to maintain your milk supply. An electric pump can be rented or purchased. This is the most efficient type of pump. Most electric pumps can pump both breasts at the same time. Manual or mini-electric pumps are less expensive and more portable, but not as efficient. Most manual pumps will pump only one breast at a time. Your health care provider or other breast-feeding expert can help you with questions about getting and using a pump that will meet your needs.

Hand expression (nothing to buy):

Hand or manual expression of breast milk is a good skill to learn even if you plan to purchase a pump. It is definitely the most portable of all methods and costs nothing. Some women express as much milk by hand as they can by using a pump. You may find it helpful for someone to demonstrate this technique for you. Ask your health care provider or breast-feeding expert for guidance.

Breast-feeding and working:

Working mothers who breast feed say that breast-feeding makes working easier.

- They have babies who are sick less often

- Night feedings are quicker

- Giving breast milk to their babies makes them feel close even when they are away at work

- They are able to continue breast-feeding at home

Let your supervisor know that you plan to continue breast-feeding when you return to work, so you can locate a clean, private area where you can pump your milk. You will need to pump on breaks and during lunch, so you will need to talk about some flexibility in your work schedule. Your breaks should not take longer than 15-20 minutes if you use a double pump. Milk can be stored in a refrigerator or a cooler with ice packs.

Expressing breast milk (EBM):

Expressed breast milk can be used to feed your infant while you're away. Your health care provider or other breast-feeding expert can help you with questions about expressing breast milk and help you to determine a plan that is best for you. You may begin expressing milk for storage after 2-3 weeks of nursing.

You can choose one or more of the following methods for expressing milk:

- Hand expression
  - This means not using a pump. Some women express as much milk by hand as they can by using a pump.
- Rent or buy and electric pump
  - This is the most efficient type of pump. If you get one that pumps both breasts at the same time, expressing takes 10-15 minutes.
- Buy a mini-electric, battery operated or manual pump
  - These are less expensive, but not as efficient as an electric pump. Most will only pump one breast at a time.

- Milk Expression Pointers

    - Always wash your hands before you begin.

    - Empty your breasts on a routine schedule to help maintain your milk supply.

    - It is helpful to express your milk on your baby(ies) nursing schedule.

    - Gently massage your breasts before expressing your breast milk.

Storing expressed breast milk:

Since many consider breast milk to be a "living substance", storage is an important thing to consider. The guidance contained in this section is supported by the Department of Health and Human Services and pertains to mothers who intend on storing their breast milk for home use. Breast milk actually has anti-bacterial properties that help it stay fresh. There are many resources available to answer any questions you might have, so just talk with your health care provider or lactation consultant.

- Guidelines

    - All milk should be dated before storing

    - The containers used should be washed in hot, soapy water and rinsed well

    - Milk may be stored in hard-sided plastic or glass containers will well-fitted tops or in freezer milk bags designed for storing human milk

    - Breast milk can be stored[3]
        - At room temperature (66°-72° F, 19°-22° C) for up to 10 hours
        - In a refrigerator (32°-39° F, 0°-4° C) for up to 8 days
        - In a freezer compartment inside a refrigerator (variable temp due to door opening frequently) for up to 2 weeks
        - In a freezer compartment with a separate door (variable temp due to door opening frequently) for up to 3 to 4 months
        - In a separate deep freeze (0° F, -19° C) for up to 6 months or longer

    - If frozen milk is defrosted in the refrigerator, it can be safely kept refrigerated for 24 hours.

    - Breast milk should not be refrozen

    - Breast milk in containers should be swirled, not shaken hard

    - Thawing breast milk containers
        - Never use the microwave to thaw breast milk
        - Thawing should take place under warm, running water

Breast-feeding after Cesarean Section:

It is very possible to breast feed after a cesarean section. Be sure to tell your health care provider of you want to do this, so that he/she can make provisions to help you. You can also write this in your birth plan. Some helpful hints include:

- Nurse as soon as possible after delivery. Many facilities are changing their routines to get your healthy baby(ies) to you within one to two hours after delivery.

- Take pain medications as needed; they won't hurt your baby and you will be more comfortable.

- Get help, especially if baby is not latching on or nursing well.

Breast-feeding Challenges:

Sore Nipples:

Studies have shown that the majority of breast-feeding women experience some nipple soreness. In about a quarter of these moms, the soreness progresses to cracking and extreme nipple pain. The most frequent causes of sore nipples is incorrect positioning.

The first two to four days after delivery, your nipples may feel tender at the beginning of a feeding as your baby's early sucking stretches your nipple and areolar tissue. If a baby is positioned well at the breast, this temporary tenderness usually diminishes once the milk lets down and then completely disappears within a day or two.

Some common treatments for sore nipples include:

- Massage your breast to encourage breast milk flow and emptying of your breast.

- Short frequent feedings are far more beneficial than long extended periods of feeding and reduces the likelihood of the infant being too vigorous at the breast and too irritable.

- Bathing a crack in the nipple in freshly expressed breast milk. This is both soothing and naturally healing.

- If you desire to use a "nipple cream," use anhydrous lanolin. This is the only cream/ ointment recommended for use on nipples.

- Learn proper positioning of your baby at your breast. Your baby should be nose to nipple, and tummy to tummy with you. The baby's chin should be just below the nipple, and the baby needs to open wide to take in a good mouthful. Never let someone shove the infant's head onto nipple until baby demonstrates signs of being ready.

- Talk to your health care provider, your certified lactation consultant or your nearest La Leche League if the above remedies don't help

Avoid:

- Placing wet tea bags on your nipples. Tannic acid in the tea can act as an astringent causing drying and cracking, rather than healing.

- Using a hair dryer or sun lamp to dry the skin.

- Most commercial preparations sold for the treatment of sore nipples. They are not useful and some may even cause harm.

Tingling Sensations:

After baby has nursed for a few minutes many (but not all) women feel a tingling sensation followed by a strong surge of milk. This is known as the "let down" response and is natural and expected. This can happen with nursing, with just seeing a baby, hearing a baby cry or even thinking about your baby. Often this let down is accompanied by leakage of milk from both breasts. To stop the milk from leaking, gently press on your nipples with a clean cloth or with your forearm. Some women wear nursing pads (without plastic liners) to help prevent leaking.

Engorgement:

You will most likely feel your breast milk come in (usually around two to six days after delivery). This is especially true if it is your first time breast-feeding. For first time moms who breast-feed, within a relatively short time period (sometimes only a few hours) your breasts become swollen, and may become painful and difficult for baby to latch on to. Thee are signs that your breasts are making the final changes necessary to make milk for your baby. This lasts only a few days at most. It is caused by blood engorgement (swelling) that comes with filling of the breast and usually goes completely away by day ten. If this is not your first baby, you probably will not experience engorgement, even though you are producing more milk now than you were at this time with your last baby. This is often perceived as decreased milk supply, but is not the case. It is just decreased discomfort so enjoy!

To help overcome engorgement try:

- Gentle breast massages: stroking the breast from the outer edges to the nipple area, especially when in a warm shower or in dependent position.

- Try warm packs followed by expressing some milk before feedings.

- If baby is having difficulty latching on, try ice only to the nipple and only for a very short period of time along with expressing milk before feeding.

- Try short frequent feedings and try not to skip any feedings.

- Start your feedings on the least sore side.

- You may use over the counter pain relief medications such as Motrin® or Tylenol®, if needed. Consult with your health care provider for the best medication for you.

Plugged ducts:

Occasionally the ducts that store milk inside your breasts can become blocked and inflamed causing a very tender spot, redness or sore lump in the breast. There are many causes including: improper positioning of the baby at your breast, too long between feedings, supplementary bottles, overuse of pacifiers, dried milk secretions covering one of the nipple openings, or wearing tight nursing bras or other restrictive clothing.

To remedy this:

- Loosen all constrictive clothing, especially your bra. Avoid under-wire bras.

- Rest often, preferably with baby in bed with you.

- Massage your breasts to help release milk from ducts prior to putting your infant to breast.

- Nurse your baby on the affected side frequently.

- Change nursing positions often to put pressure on different ducts.

- Clean nipples to ensure no milk is blocking the ducts.

- Make sure the sore breast gets emptied of milk either through baby or expression by hand or pump.

- Soaking the sore breast in a basin of warm water may help.

- DO NOT STOP OR SLOW DOWN ON FEEDINGS as this can add to the problem.

Since plugged ducts can lead to infection, it is important to remedy the situation as quickly as possible.

Breast Infection:

If you notice the signs of a plugged duct becoming more severe and combined with fever or flu-like symptoms, you could have a breast infection called mastitis. You need to treat a breast infection *immediately.* Continue breast-feeding! Start with applying heat to he affected area, breast massage to help empty your breast and try to get plenty of rest. If these steps don't resolve the symptoms within 24 hours call your health care provider without delay. You will most likely be treated with antibiotics and mild pain relievers. While taking the medications you will also need plenty of rest, increased fluid intake, moist heat applications to your breasts and frequent nursing beginning with the infected breast. Delaying treatment could result in developing a breast abscess. Let your health care provider or certified lactation consultant know if you have had a previous history of mastitis.

- Vary nursing positions to avoid pressure on the same ducts.

- Clean nipples to ensure no milk is blocking the ducts.

- DO NOT stop or slow down on feedings.

Some Web Site References:

- U.S. Department of Health and Human Services Office on Women's Health: www.4woman.gov/Breast-feeding

- La Leche League International: www.lalecheleague.org

- San Diego County Breast-feeding Coalition: www.breast-feeding.org/

References used in this Section
1. *Weimer, Jon P. Breast-feeding: Health and Economic Issues, Food Review, Vol 22, Issue 2, May-August 1999.*
2. *U.S. Department of Health and Human Services. HHS Blueprint for Action on Breast-feeding, Washington, D.C. US Department of Health and Human Services, Office on Women's Health, 2000.*
3. *La Leche League International. Human Milk Storage Information. www.lalecheleague.org/FAQ/milkstorage.html, Feb 2003*

Bottle Feeding

Whether you decide to breast-feed, bottle feed expressed milk, or formula, you will see that feeding time is an important time for you and your baby to get to know and love each other. Always use feeding time to share comfort and closeness.

Do not give your baby anything but breast milk or iron fortified formula until instructed by your healthcare provider. Any commercial infant formula is adequate for normal infant growth. In the first months, the baby will take 2-4 ounces every 3-4 hours. Follow the instructions on the can carefully. Some formulas are "ready to feed" and don't need added water, others are concentrated and have to be diluted. If your baby has problems with the brand of formula you are using, contact your health care provider before switching to another formula.

Always check the expiration date and the lot number on the formula cans. Do not use dented, leaking, or damaged containers of formula, since these could have bacteria in them.

- If you are using tap water to mix the formula, let the water run for several minutes before you add it to the container. You do not have to boil the water. Do not keep uncovered formula cans in the refrigerator.

- Warm the milk by setting the bottle in warm water (never in the microwave).

- Once you have warmed the bottle (or removed it from the refrigerator), it should be given immediately. Hold the baby with his/her head higher than his body and touch the nipple to his lips. Let baby open his/her mouth to take the nipple. Do not force the nipple in.

- Never prop the bottle or put the baby to bed with a bottle. This can lead to choking and it causes tooth decay.

- Let the baby decide when he/she has had enough. If baby refuses the bottle, try burping. If baby still refuses to eat after burping, stop until the next feeding.

- A healthy baby will stop eating when full.

- Throw away the formula left in the bottle from that feeding. Rinse the bottle and nipple after use with cold water. It makes clean up easier.

- Bottles and nipples can be washed in the dishwasher or in hot, soapy water.

Bottle feeding Supplies:

- Baby bottles and caps

- Nipples

- Bottle and nipple brush

- Measuring cups

Safety Tips for Baby

- Sleeping tips:
    - Always place baby on his or her back to sleep.
    - Never give a baby a bottle in the bed.
    - Bedding should be firm and snugly fit the crib.
    - Crib slats should be no farther apart than 2 inches (6 cm).
    - Keep crib away from drapery and blind cords, heaters, wall decorations, and other potential hazards.
    - Never use a pillow in the crib.
    - Keep mobiles and other crib toys out of baby's reach.
- Warm temperatures (not hot) for baby.
- Never prop a bottle or leave baby alone with a bottle.
- Don't put your baby in an infant seat on the counter or table.
- Never leave a baby unattended in any water. One inch of water is enough for a baby to drown in.
- Keep baby's air smoke-free .
- Never microwave a baby's bottle.
- Shake or stir all bottles and food before giving to baby.
- Never hang anything on baby's stroller-it can cause it to tip over.
- Breast-feed if at all possible.
- Never leave baby alone on any surface above the floor, not even for a few seconds.
- Infant walkers are NOT recommended due to safety problems.
- All rattles and teethers need to be one piece and larger than 1 inch.
- Never attach a pacifier around baby's neck.
- Make sure all smoke detectors are in working order.
- Keep water heater on 120° F or "low" setting.
- Don't carry hot liquids or cook when carrying your baby.

Analgesia
Medication used to reduce your ability to feel pain.

Anemia
Condition in which your blood has decreased oxygen carrying ability as a result of low number of cells (hemotocrit) or a decrease in hemoglobin. Adequate intake of iron in the diet can help prevent iron deficiency anemia.

Anesthesia
Medication that causes a loss of feeling or sensation.

Amniocentesis
With the help of an ultrasound, a needle is inserted through your abdomen into your uterus and a small sample of amniotic fluid from the amniotic sac is taken to test for several genetic problems, as well as, for your baby's lung maturity. This test is usually performed between 16 and 20 weeks on women with risks for genetic problems.

Amniotic Sac
Fluid filled, thin-walled sac in which the fetus develops that is often called the "bag of waters." This sac protects the baby from injury and regulates its temperature.

Antepartum
The period of time from conception to labor.

Antibody
Substance in blood that is produced in response to foreign protein to develop immunity.

Antigen
Substance that can induce an immune response and cause the production of an antibody.

Anus
Opening of the rectum located behind the vagina.

Asymptomatic Bacteriuria (ASB)
Bacteria in urine that does not cause any signs or symptoms of an infection. Occurs in 2-7% of pregnant women and can lead to complications in pregnancy such as pre-term delivery and low birth weight babies. You are checked for this by a urine test at your first visit.

Bloody Show
Bloody discharge of mucus, which forms in the cervix and is expelled right before or at the beginning of labor.

Braxton-Hicks contractions (false labor)
Irregular tightening of the uterus you may feel as your body prepares for delivery; may be felt weeks before labor.

Cervix
The neck or opening of the uterus through which the baby passes during the birth process. The cervix projects into the vagina and is made up of mainly fibrous tissue and muscle. Labor contractions result in effacement (thinning or shortening) and dilatation (opening) of the cervix.

Chlamydia
Sexually transmitted disease that can cause pelvic inflammatory disease, infertility, and problems during pregnancy. This is tested for at your 10-12 week appointment through a speculum (pelvic) exam and can be cured with antibiotics.

Chorionic Villus Sampling (CVS)
This procedure tests for the same genetic problems as an amniocentesis but it is performed earlier in your pregnancy (usually between your 10th and 13th week). With the help of an ultrasound to see inside your uterus, a needle is inserted through your abdomen and into your uterus to take a small sample of cells from the amniotic lining for testing. There are some risks involved with this procedure such as miscarriages (more than with an amniocentesis) and possible limb defects (especially when done before 10 weeks pregnant).

Contraction
The shortening and tightening of the uterus, which results in the dilation (opening) and effacement (thinning or shortening) of the cervix.

Crowning
The bulging out of the perineum as the baby's head or presenting part presses against it at time of delivery.

Cystic Fibrosis
A genetic disease that is inherited from both parents and causes life-long illness affecting breathing and digestion. A blood test can tell if you or the baby's father carries this trait. If both of you carry the Cystic Fibrosis trait, your baby has a 25% chance of acquiring the disease. Usually the woman is tested first; then, if positive, the father of the baby will be tested. You should sign a consent form to have this test performed.

Doppler
Device that looks like a stethoscope that allows your baby's heartbeat to be heard through ear pieces or speaker.

Down's Syndrome (Trisomy 21)
Genetic disorder caused by the presence of an extra chromosome and characterized by mental retardation, abnormal features of the face, and medical problems such as heart defects. Chances of your baby carrying this disorder increase with increasing age of the mom. This can be tested for between 15 and 20 weeks of your pregnancy with the Maternal Serum Analyte Screen.

Embryo
The developing organism from about two weeks after fertilization to the end of the seventh or eighth week.

Epidural
Type of regional anesthesia in which medication is inserted into the spinal space through a small plastic tube.

Estriol

Hormone made by the placenta and the fetal liver. The estriol level is measured as part of the Maternal Serum Analyte Screen.

Fetal Distress

A condition in which the baby is deprived of oxygen that can be seen by changes in the pattern of the baby's heartbeat.

Fetus

A developing baby in the uterus after the seventh to ninth week of gestation until birth.

Forceps

An instrument placed on both sides of the baby's head, while in the birth canal, to gently pull the baby out if needed.

Fundal Height

Measurement from the pubic bone to the top of the uterus or fundus. Routinely used to measure the growth of the baby in the uterus.

Gestation

Development of the new baby within the uterus from conception to birth.

Gonorrhea (GC, the clap)

Sexually transmitted disease that may lead to pelvic inflammatory disease, infertility, and arthritis. It is tested at your 10 to 12 week visit by taking a sample of your vaginal secretions. It can be treated with antibiotics.

Group B Streptococcus (GBS)

A bacteria commonly found in the vagina and the rectum. GBS grows in the vagina or rectum in about 10-40% of women and rarely causes symptoms. In pregnancy, it can increase your chances of premature delivery, premature rupture of membranes, infection of your amniotic fluid and serious infection in your baby. A different type of streptococcus bacteria causes the condition known as "Strep throat." To find out if you have any GBS, vaginal and rectal secretions are collected between the 35th and 37th week of your pregnancy. If you are found to have GBS, antibiotics during your labor are given to protect your baby from these bacteria.

Hematocrit

Blood test that measures the number of cells in your blood. This test shows whether you are anemic (low in iron).

Hemoglobin

Blood test that measures your oxygen carrying ability of your blood and gives information on whether you are anemic (low in iron).

Hepatitis B Virus

Attacks and damages the liver, causing inflammation, cirrhosis, and chronic hepatitis that can lead to cancer. This is tested for at your first prenatal visit. It can be transmitted to your baby and infect the baby. If you think you have been exposed to this you will be tested, and given a vaccine. If you have the disease, you will receive treatment that greatly reduces your baby's risk of getting the disease.

Human Immunodeficiency Virus (HIV)
Attacks certain cells of the body's immune system and causes acquired immunodeficiency syndrome (AIDS). There is a blood test which can be drawn at your first prenatal visit to determine if you have the disease. If you test positive, you can receive treatment that can greatly reduce the baby's risk of getting the disease.

Human Papilloma Virus (HPV)
Sexually transmitted disease characterized by soft wart like growths on the genitalia. Commonly referred to as genital warts. Pregnancy can cause warts to increase in size or appear for the first time. Usually no treatment is needed and they go away on their own after the delivery. If the warts grow very large and obstruct the birth canal, treatment and/or cesarean section may be needed. HPV infection can also be without symptoms and only show up years later as a result of a pap test. Certain strains of HPV have been linked to increased cervical cancer.

Induction of Labor
Artificially cause labor to start by rupturing the bag of waters or giving medications such as pitocin or prostaglandin.

Iso-immunization
Occurs when an Rh (D-)Negative mom develops antibodies to her baby's Rh (D)Positive blood. RhoGAM injection prevents this from occurring to protect the baby.

Labor
The series of uterine contractions that dilate (open) the cervix for birth.

Libido
Sexual desire.

Maternal Serum Analyte Screen
Group of blood tests, also known as a Tripple Screen, that check for substances linked with certain birth defects such as Down's syndrome (Trisomy 21), neural tube defects, Edwards Syndrome (Trisomy 18) and other related birth defects. The test is done during the 15th to 20th week of your pregnancy. If you get an abnormal test result, this result will be further checked with an ultrasound and possibly an amniocentesis. This test has many false positives.

Maturation
Achievement of full development or growth.

Meconium
Baby's first bowel movement, usually passed after birth. When it is passed before birth, it stains the amniotic fluid and is possibly a sign of distress. When this occurs, it is referred to as meconium staining.

Neonatology
Branch of medicine that specializes in the high-risk newborn.

Neural Tube Defects (NTDs)
Birth defects that result from improper development of the brain, spinal cord, or their coverings. This can be tested for at around 16 weeks in your pregnancy with a Maternal Serum Analyte Screen blood test.

Pap Test
Cells are taken from the cervix and vagina and examined to check for abnormalities that may lead to cervical cancer.

Perinatologist
Obstetrician who specializes in high-risk pregnancies.

Perineum
The surface area between the vagina and anus in females; between the scrotum and anus in males.

Placenta (afterbirth)
An organ of pregnancy attached to the wall of the uterus where oxygen, nutrients, and waste exchange takes place between the mother and fetus. It delivers within 30 minutes of the baby's birth.

Postpartum
The 6-week period following childbirth.

Pre-Eclampsia – see Pregnancy-Induced Hypertension

Pregnancy-Induced Hypertension (PIH)
A condition also known as pre-eclampsia or toxemia. You will be monitored for this condition throughout you pregnancy with blood pressure checks at each visit and lab work, if needed.

RhoGAM
A medication given through an injection (shot) at 28 weeks to Rh (D-) negative women to prevent iso-immunization. If baby is Rh (D) positive, the new mother will receive another injection after delivery.

Rubella Test
Blood test taken at your first visit to see if you are protected against Rubella (German measles). If you are not protected against this disease, your health care provider will discuss your need to avoid anyone who might have the disease.

Sexually Transmitted Diseases (STD)
An infection spread by sexual contact: Gonorrhea, Syphilis, Chlamydia, HIV, HPV, Hepatitis B and Trichomonas.

Syphilis
Sexually transmitted disease that is caused by an organism called Treponema Palladium; it may cause major health problems or death in its later stages. The blood test is taken at your first prenatal visit.

Toxemia – see Pregnancy-Induced Hypertension

Triple Screen - see Maternal Serum Analyte Screen

Ultrasound
Through the use of sound waves, this machine gives a live black and white picture of your baby. Routinely performed in the Military Treatment Facilities at 16-20 weeks to screen for problems and determine your due date.

Umbilical Cord
A fetal structure that connects the fetus to the placenta; contains two arteries and one vein to provide blood flow between the fetus and placenta.

Uterus (womb)

The hollow muscular organ in which a unborn baby develops and grows. The muscles of the uterus contract during labor and help push the baby out through the vagina.

Vacuum Extraction

Suctions baby out of the birth canal by applying a metal or plastic cup to baby's head and applying suction from a wall or portable suction machine.

Vagina

Lower part of the birth canal behind the bladder and in front of the rectum.

VDRL (Venereal Disease Research Laboratory)

Blood test taken at your first visit that screens for Syphilis, a sexually transmitted disease. If your test is positive, you will be offered treatment and the risks to your baby will be discussed.

Ancillary Staff
Staff members who work in the clinics to assist you. They may be clerical support, registered nurses, licensed vocational nurses, medical assistants, and corpsmen. They work to assist with your needs as their qualifications allow.

Anesthesiologist
A physician specialized in pain relief.

Certified Nurse Midwife (CNM)
A registered nurse with a Master's degree and certification by the American College of Nurse Midwives. Nurse midwifery practice is the independent management of women's health care that focuses on pregnancy, childbirth, the postpartum period, newborn care, family planning, and the gynecological needs of women with an emphasis on education and health promotion.

Family Nurse Practitioner (FNP)
A registered nurse with advanced degrees specializing in the treatment and care for patients of all ages. FNPs can provide prenatal care and coordinate care with a physician for delivery of the baby.

Family Practice (FP) Physician
A physician specially trained to provide medical care to patients of all ages, diagnose and treat all illnesses. They provide prenatal care and delivery services.

OB/GYN Physician
A physician specialized in the area of Obstetrics and Gynecology. He or she can provide routine or complicated care and can provide surgical services as needed.

Neonatologist
A pediatrician specialized in the care of newborns.

Nurse Anesthetist
A nurse specialized in pain relief.

Pediatrician
A physician specialized in the care of infants and children.

Resident
A physician who has graduated from medical school and is in training at a teaching hospital.

Women's Health Nurse Practitioner
A registered nurse with an advanced degree specializing in the care of women throughout their life-span, including prenatal, contraception, and menopause. They can provide routine prenatal care and postpartum care, with an emphasis on education and health promotion.